# Plastic
# Survival Guide
# to Trauma



**Amir Nakhdjevani, Richard Baker and Hootan Ahmadi**

*The* ROYAL
SOCIETY *of*
MEDICINE
PRESS *Limited*

Published by the Royal Society of Medicine Press Ltd
1 Wimpole Street, London W1G 0AE, UK
Tel: +44 (0)20 7290 2921
Fax: +44 (0)20 7290 2929
Email: publishing@rsm.ac.uk
Website: www.rsmpress.co.uk



**British Library Cataloguing in Publication Data**
A catalogue record for this book is available from the British Library

ISBN 978-1-85315-770-7

Distribution in Europe and Rest of World:

Marston Book Services Ltd
PO Box 269
Abingdon
Oxon OX14 4YN, UK
Tel: +44 (0)1235 465500
Fax: +44 (0)1235 465555
Email: direct.order@marston.co.uk

Distribution in the USA and Canada:

Royal Society of Medicine Press Ltd
c/o BookMasters Inc
30 Amberwood Parkway
Ashland, OH 44805, USA
Tel: +1 800 247 6553/+1 800 266 5564
Fax: +1 419 281 6883
Email: order@bookmasters.com

Distribution in Australia and New Zealand:

Elsevier Australia
30-52 Smidmore Street
Marrikville NSW 2204, Australia
Tel: +61 2 9517 8999
Fax: +61 2 9517 2249
Email: service@elsevier.com.au

Designed and typeset by Phoenix Photosetting, Chatham, Kent

Printed and bound in Netherlands by Alfabase

# Contents

# Acknowledgements

For reviewing parts of the manuscript we would like to thank the following Consultant Plastic Surgeons: Mr Baljit Dheansa, Mr Adriaan Grobbelaar, Mr David Martin, Mr John Pereira; and Consultant Anaethetist: Dr Chetan Patel.

AN, RB, HA

I would like to dedicate this book firstly to my parents for their love and support throughout my like. (Barri va Baba firouz doostetoon darm.) I would like to thank my wife, Rosie, for putting up with my daily long hours and supporting me in my career.

Thanks to Kieran Dawson for inspiring me to pursue a career in surgery and for guiding me through the years. You have given me the wisdom of your experience and been a support in my life. Thanks to my friend Vasu Karri the Professor and my guide. Thanks to Chetan Patel the coolest and the best anaesthetist I know. Working with Chet is fun, educational and inspiring. Thanks Chet for your support, friendship and the three minutes warning!

Last, but not least, John Pereira who is my consultant, mentor, guide and a true friend for life. Words cannot describe your qualities. You have taught me so much that thanks alone is not enough. I appreciate the time and effort you have invested in me. Your have set the standards in everything I do.

AN

I dedicate this book to my parents

RB

John Collins for my first opportunity in medicine; Peta Longstaff for kick-starting my career; Martin Kelly, for your help, guidance and ever-present advice – thanks boss; Donald Dewar and John Simmons for initiating my surgical tuition; David Floyd and Simon Withey for my first Plastics exposure; Inaki Bovill, Patrick Roberts, Carlos Cobiella, and Barbara Jemec for their help, advice and friendship; Effie Katsarma for guiding me in my first registrar job.

My extended family in medicine – Abtin Alvand, Akbar de' Medici, Alex Woollard, Ali Rismani, Alice Danczak, Andrew Gogbashian, Dave Gill, Ghias Bhattee, Henry Colaco, Karan Kapoor, Leo Monzon, Mo Akhavani and Roger Crystal.

Lucian Ion – my guide, my mentor, and my friend. Thank you for everything, the list is too long.

My loving family – Arshia, Flore, Mahboob, Maman Joon, Mamani, Mehrdad, Naghi, Nima, Raha and the rest of my family and friends outside medicine.

HA

# Introduction

This book covers immediate management of hand trauma as well as other common emergencies and ward problems seen in plastic and reconstructive surgery. It is particularly aimed at junior doctors who are new to plastic surgery, but it is also relevant to junior doctors in the specialties of general practice, emergency medicine, and orthopaedics and trauma.

This book is not a textbook but a guide to the safe immediate management of plastic surgery patients until definitive treatment can be undertaken. It is written by junior plastic surgeons for junior plastic surgeons and tells the reader exactly what they need to know and do when they are on the ward, in the emergency department or taking referrals. This book will give new plastic surgeons knowledge at the start of the job, which, until now, could be acquired only 'on the job'.

We hope you find this a dependable guide in those first few hectic weeks.

# 1 Hand trauma

Hand trauma will form the bulk of your on-call work. Management is pretty much the same in all cases: wound irrigation, elevation, antibiotics, tetanus vaccination and appropriate surgery. The main decisions are when to admit the patient, when to operate and which anaesthetic to arrange.

Conditions to be wary of are ischaemia, dislocations, replantable amputations, infection and crush injuries (compartment syndrome). These represent the scenarios in which you need to act urgently and inform your registrar. These and other injuries will be described in this section.

# Anatomy of the upper limb

The hand is one of the most complex structures in nature, and this complexity enables remarkable dexterity. A complete anatomical description of the hand is beyond the scope of this book; however, it is important to understand the fundamental basics to allow a structured assessment of the injuries we aim to address. Movements take place through coordination of the small muscles of the hand as well as the muscles extending from the forearm, so we will consider these muscles in our unveiling of the anatomy.

## Flexor compartment of the arm

The flexor compartment of the arm can be classified broadly into superficial, intermediate and deep compartments (Table 1.1). Figure 1.1 shows a layered, illustrated dissection of the forearm muscles superimposed on a photograph of an arm to allow you to orientate yourself when assessing forearm injuries.

## Lateral compartment of the arm

The lateral compartment consists of two muscles supplied by the radial nerve. Both of these muscles originate from the supracondylar ridge of the humerus. Table 1.2 illustrates the muscles of the lateral compartment of the forearm.

## Extensor compartment of the arm

The extensor compartment of the arm is supplied solely by the radial nerve and can be subdivided into superficial and deep compartments (Table 1.3). Muscles of the extensor compartment of the forearm are shown in Figure 1.2.

## Small muscles of the hand

Numerous muscles in the hand allow us to perform tasks with great dexterity. Table 1.4 illustrates these muscles and their subcategorization. Figure 1.3 illustrates the dorsal and Figure 1.4 the palmar interossei of the hand. Note their

**Table 1.1** Characteristics of the components of the flexor compartment of the forearm.

| Compartment | Name | Origin | Insertion | Nerve | Action |
|---|---|---|---|---|---|
| Superficial | • Pronator teres | • Medial humeral epicondyle<br>• Coranoid process of ulna | • Lateral aspect of shaft of radius | • Median nerve | • Pronation and flexion of forearm |
| | • Flexor carpi radialis | • Medial humeral epicondyle | • Base of second and third metacarpal bones | • Median nerve | • Flexes and abducts hand at wrist |
| | • Palmaris longus | • Medial humeral epicondyle | • Flexor retinaculum and palmar aponeurosis | • Median nerve | • Flexes hand at wrist |
| | • Flexor carpi ulnaris | • Medial humeral epicondyle<br>• Olecranon process of ulna | • Pisiform via pisohamate and pisometacarpal ligaments into hamate and base of metacarpal bone | • Ulnar nerve | • Flexes and adducts hand at wrist |
| Intermediate | • Flexor digitorum superficialis | • Medial humeral epicondyle<br>• Coranoid process of ulna<br>• Shaft of radius | • Two heads unite<br>• Gives rise to four tendons that pass under flexor retinaculum<br>• Hand: tendons divide into slips, unite, divide again and insert into sides of middle phalanx | • Median nerve | • Flexes middle phalanx<br>• Aids in flexing proximal phalanx |
| Deep | • Flexor pollicis longus | • Anterior surface or radius<br>• Interosseous membrane | • Base of distal phalanx of thumb | • Median nerve | • Flexion of distal phalanx of thumb |
| | • Flexor digitorum profundus | • Anterior and medial surface of ulna<br>• Interosseous membrane | • Divides into four tendons that pass through tendons of flexor digitorum superficialis and insert into base of distal phalanx | • Medial half: ulnar nerve<br>• Lateral half: median nerve | • Flexion of distal phalanx of fingers |
| | • Pronator quadratus | • Lower anterior shaft of ulna | • Lower anterior shaft of radius | • Median nerve | • Pronates at distal radioulnar joint |

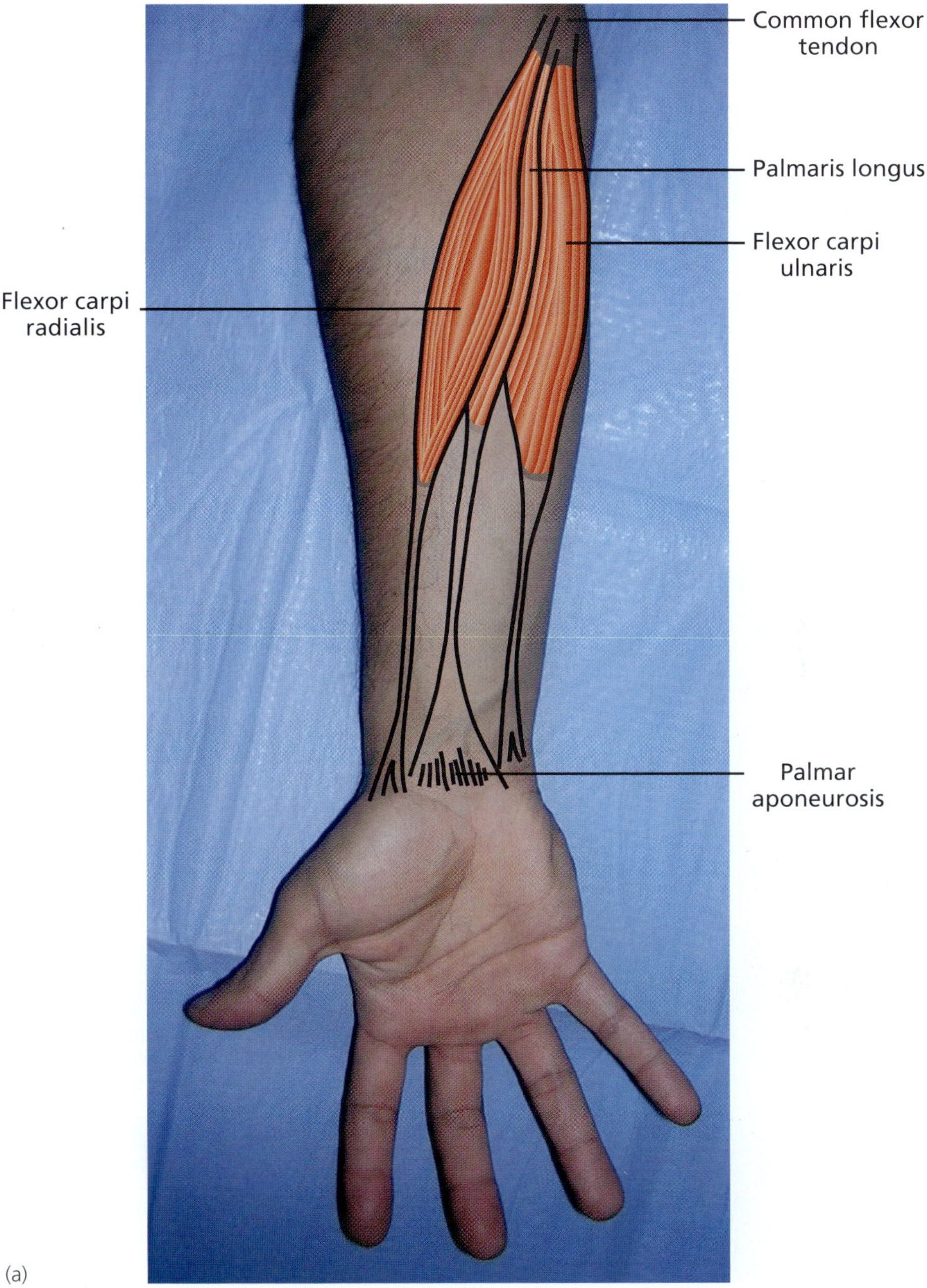


(a)

**Figure 1.1** Muscles of the flexor compartment of the forearm: (a) superficial flexor compartment (*continued*)

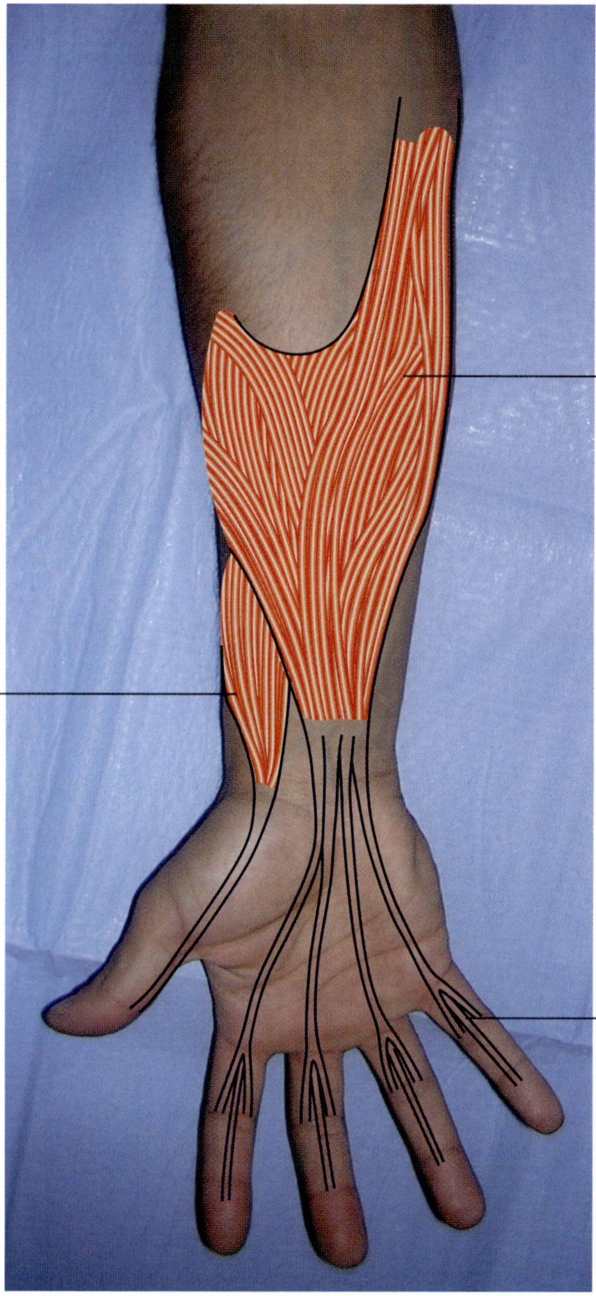


(b)

**Figure 1.1** (*continued*) Muscles of the flexor compartment of the forearm: (b) intermediate flexor compartments (*continued*)

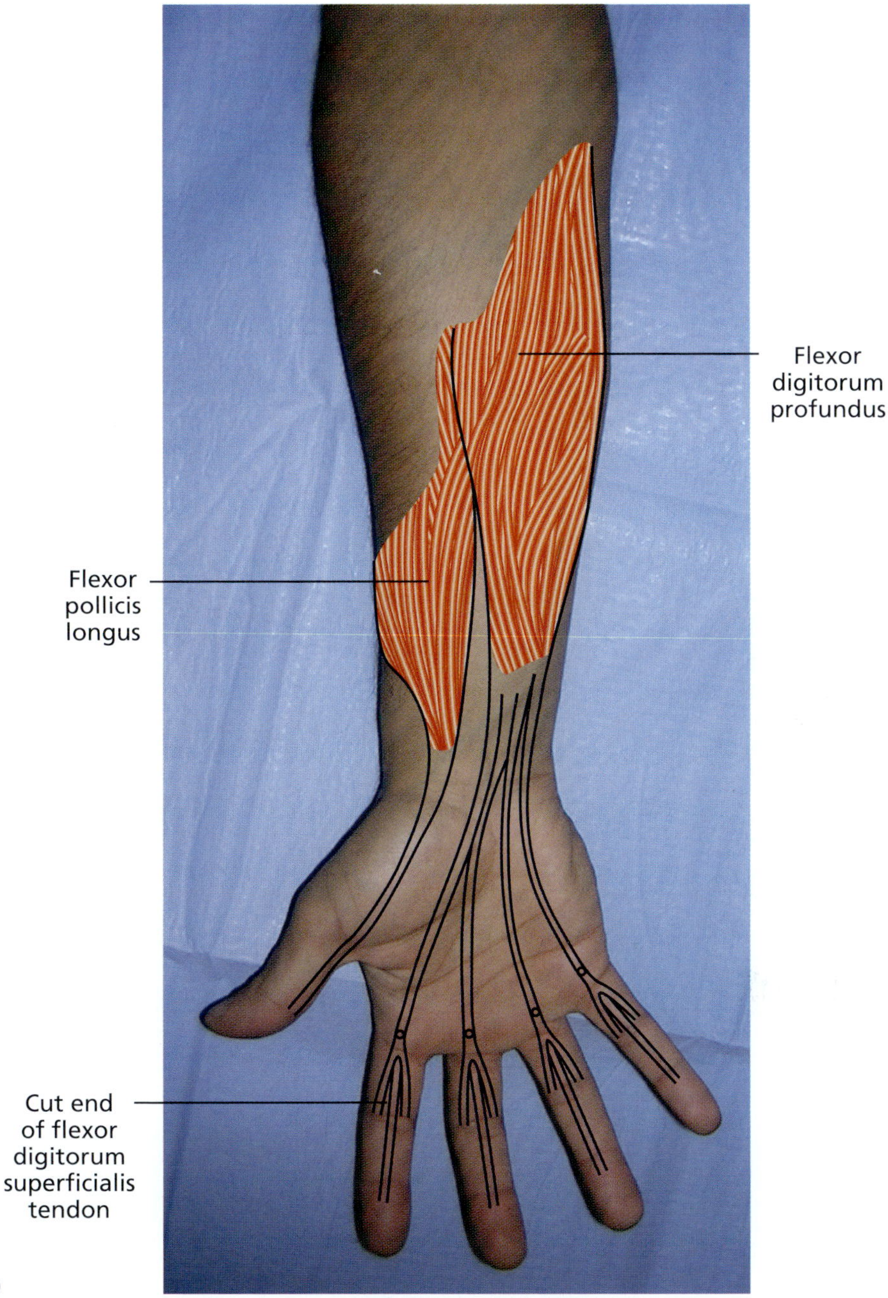


(c)

**Figure 1.1** (*continued*) Muscles of the flexor compartment of the forearm: (c) deep flexor compartment

**Table 1.2** Characteristics of the components of the lateral compartment of the forearm.

| Name | Origin | Insertion | Nerve | Action |
|---|---|---|---|---|
| Brachioradialis | • Supracondylar ridge of humerus | • Styloid process of radius | • Radial | • Flexes forearm<br>• Assist in pronation |
| Extensor carpi radialis longus | • Supracondylar ridge of humerus | • Base of second metacarpal | • Radial | • Extends and abducts hand |

**Table 1.3** Characteristics of the components of the extensor compartment of the forearm.

| Compartment | Name | Origin | Insertion | Nerve | Action |
|---|---|---|---|---|---|
| Superficial | • Extensor carpi radialis brevis | • Lateral humeral epicondyle | • Base of third metacarpal | • Radial nerve | • Extends and abducts hand |
| | • Extensor digitorum | • Lateral humeral epicondyle | • Divides into four tendons under extensor retinaculum<br>• Tendons of little, ring and middle finger connect by fibrous band<br>• Tendon of index finger joined on medial side by tendon of extensor digiti minimi<br>• Dorsal aspect of fingers: tendons widen to form extensor expansion<br>• Central part is inserted into base of middle phalanx<br>• Two lateral parts insert into base of distal phalanx | • Radial nerve | • Extends metacarpophalangeal joints<br>• Assist in extending proximal interphalangeal joint and distal interphalangeal joint |
| | • Extensor digiti minimi | • Lateral humeral epicondyle | • Divides into two slips inserted into extensor expansion of little finger | • Radial nerve | • Extends metacarpophalangeal joint of little finger |
| | • Extensor carpi ulnaris | • Lateral humeral epicondyle | • Posterior surface of base of fifth metacarpal | • Radial nerve | • Extends and adducts hand at wrist |
| | • Anconeus | • Lateral humeral epicondyle | • Lateral surface of olecranon process of ulna | • Radial nerve | • Extends elbow |
| Deep | • Supinator | • Lateral humeral epicondyle | • Winds around neck of radius inserted into posterior, lateral and anterior surface of neck and shaft of radius | • Radial nerve | • Supinator at proximal radioulnar joint |

(contd. overleaf)

**Table 1.3** (continued)

| Compartment | Name | Origin | Insertion | Nerve | Action |
|---|---|---|---|---|---|
| Deep (contd.) | • Abductor pollicis longus | • Posterior shaft of ulna and radius | • Base of first metacarpal bone | • Radial nerve | • Abducts and extends thumb at carpometacarpal joint |
| | • Extensor pollicis brevis | • Posterior shaft of ulna and radius | • Base of proximal phalanx of thumb | • Radial nerve | • Extends metacarpophalangeal joint of thumb |
| | • Extensor pollicis longus | • Posterior shaft of ulna and radius | • Posterior surface of base of distal phalanx of thumb | • Radial nerve | • Extends distal phalanx of thumb |
| | • Extensor indicis | • Posterior shaft of ulna and radius | • Extensor expansion of index finger | • Radial nerve | • Extends metacarpophalangeal joint of index finger |

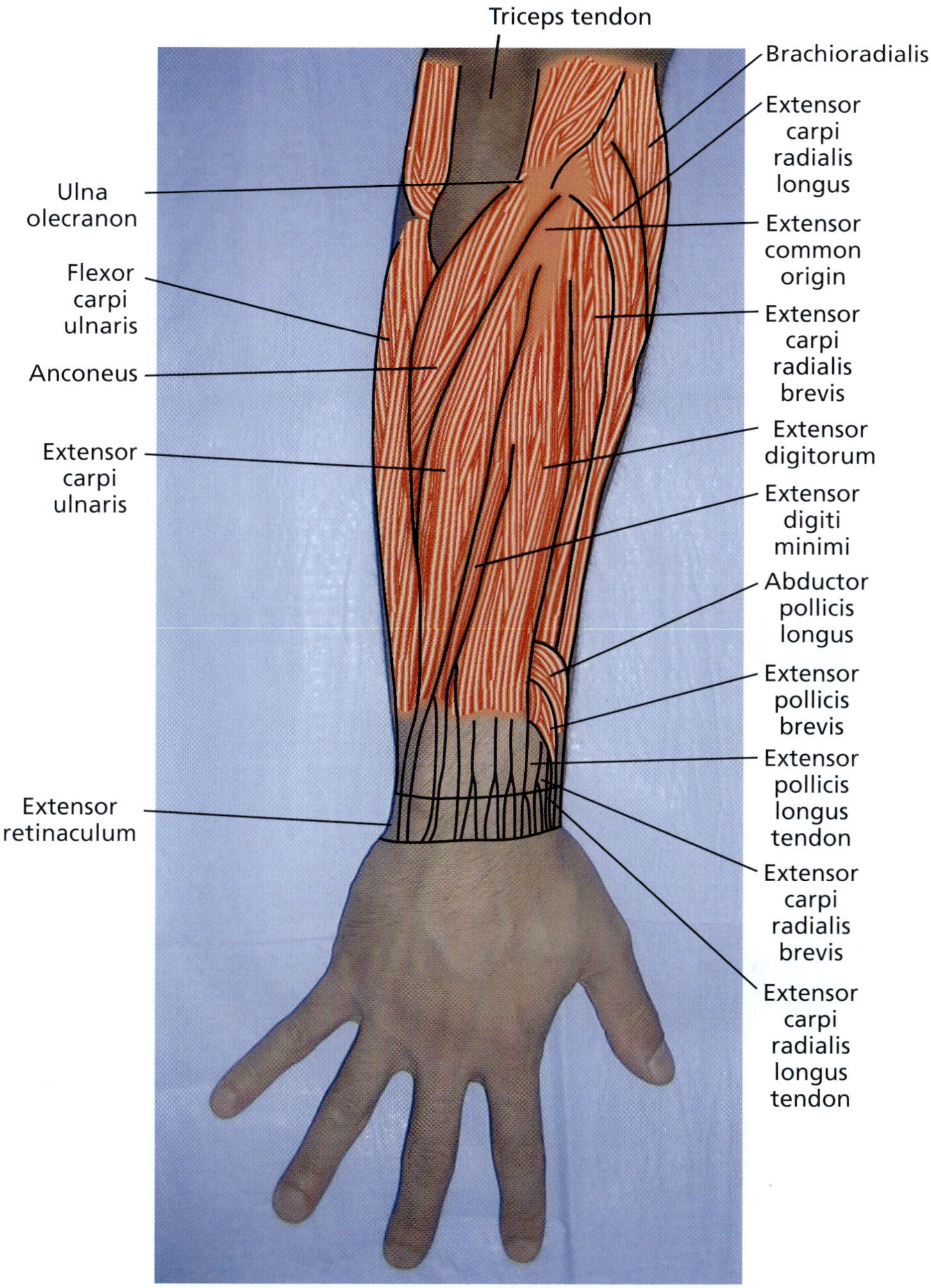


**Figure 1.2** Extensor compartment of the forearm

**Table 1.4** Characteristics of the small muscles of the hand.

| Compartment | Name | Origin | Insertion | Nerve | Action |
|---|---|---|---|---|---|
| Hand | • Lumbricals (four in number) | • Tendons of flexor digitorum profundus | • Lateral side of corresponding extensor expansion | • Lateral 2 – median nerve<br>• Medial 2 – ulnar nerve | • Assisted by interossei, flex metacarpophalangeal joint and extend interphalangeal joint |
| Interossei (eight in total) | | | • Occupy space between metacarpal bone bones | • Dorsal are larger and have two heads<br>• Palmar and smaller and have one head | |
| | • Palmar interossei | • Medial side of 1st, 2nd, 3rd and 4th metacarpal bones, respectively | • 1st – medial side of base of proximal phalanx of thumb<br>• 2nd – medial side of base of proximal phalanx of index finger<br>• 3rd – lateral side of base of proximal phalanx of ring finger<br>• 4th – lateral side of base of proximal phalanx of little finger | • Ulnar nerve | • Adduct fingers towards centre of third finger at metacarpophalangeal joint<br>• Flexes metacarpophalangeal joint and extends interphalangeal joint |
| | • Dorsal interossei | • Sides of 1st and 2nd, 2nd and 3rd, 3rd and 4th, and 4th and 5th metacarpal bones | • 1st – lateral side of base of proximal phalanx of index finger<br>• 2nd – lateral side of base of proximal phalanx of middle finger<br>• 3rd – medial side of base of proximal phalanx of middle finger<br>• 4th – medial side of base of proximal phalanx of ring finger | • Ulnar nerve | • Abduct fingers away from middle finger at metacarpophalangeal joints, extends interphalangeal joints |

**Table 1.4** (continued)

| Compartment | Name | Origin | Insertion | Nerve | Action |
|---|---|---|---|---|---|
| Thumb | • Abductor pollicis brevis | • Scaphoid<br>• Trapezium<br>• Flexor retinaculum | • Base of proximal phalanx of thumb with flexor pollicis brevis | • Median nerve | • Abducts thumb at carpo-metacarpal joint and metacarpophalangeal joint |
| | • Flexor pollicis brevis | • Flexor retinaculum | • Lateral aspect of base of proximal phalanx of thumb with abductor pollicis brevis | • Median nerve | • Flexes thumb at metacarpophalangeal joint |
| | • Opponens pollicis | • Flexor retinaculum | • Lateral border of shaft of first metacarpal bone | • Median nerve | • Pulls thumb medially and forward |
| | • Abductor pollicis | • Oblique head: base of 2nd and 3rd metacarpals and joining carpal bones<br>• Transverse head: shaft of 3rd metacarpal bone | • Heads converge and inserted with 1st palmar interossei into medial side of base of proximal phalanx of thumb | • Ulnar nerve | • Adduction of thumb at carpometacarpal and metacarpophalangeal joint |
| Little finger | • Abductor digiti minimi | • Pisiform | • Base of proximal phalanx of little finger | • Ulnar nerve | • Abducts little finger at metacarpophalangeal joint |
| | • Flexor digiti minimi | • Flexor retinaculum | • Base of proximal phalanx of little finger | • Ulnar nerve | • Flexes little finger at metacarpophalangeal joint |
| | • Opponens digiti minimi | • Flexor retinaculum | • Medial border of 5th metacarpal bone | • Ulnar nerve | • Rotation of 5th metacarpal<br>• Assists in flexion of carpometacarpal bone |

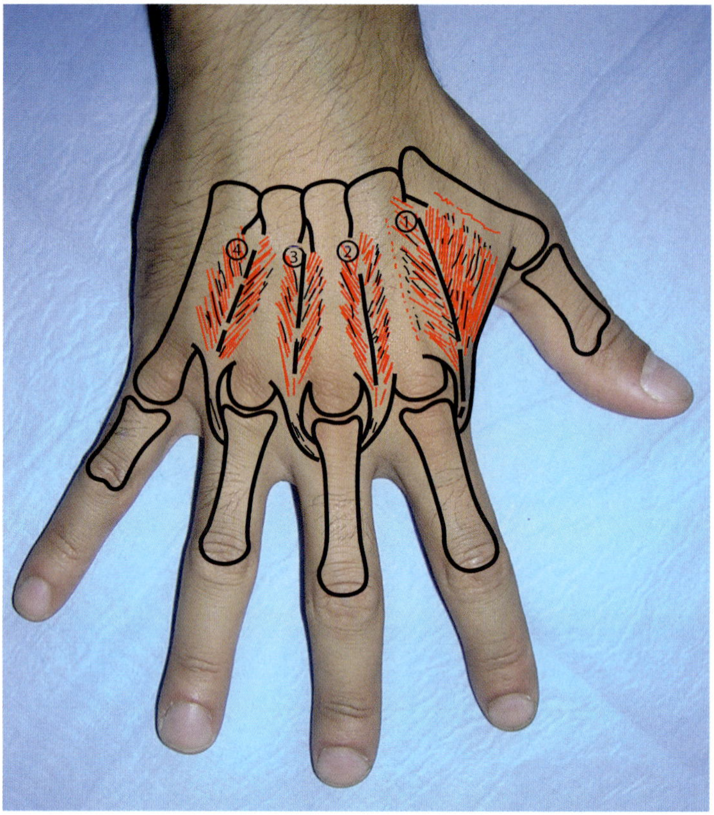


**Figure 1.3** Dorsal interossei (numbered 1 to 4)

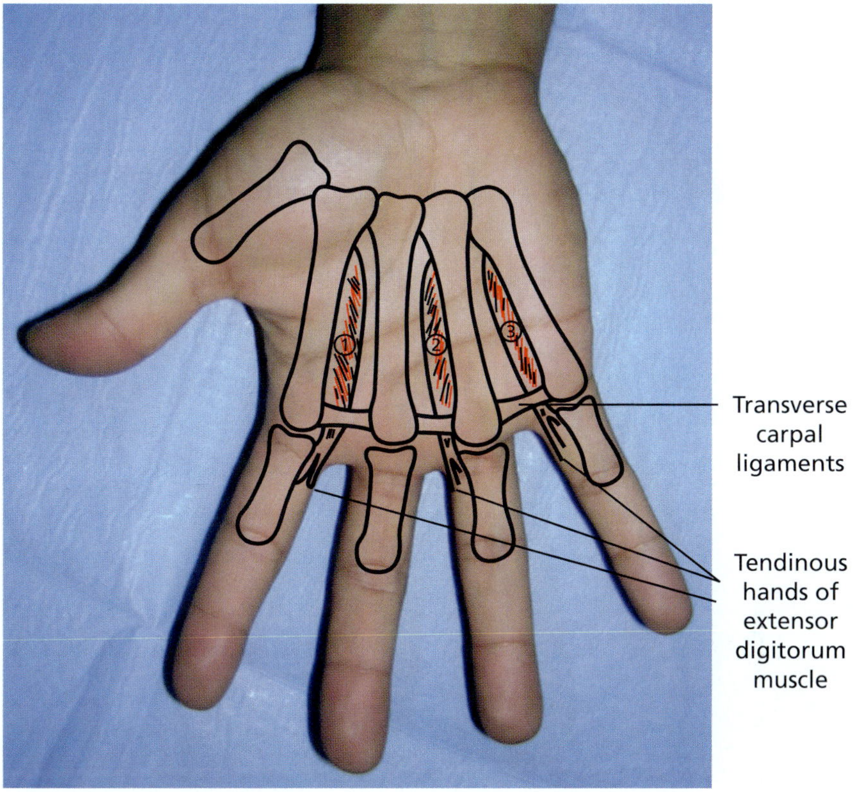


**Figure 1.4** Palmar interossei

origins and insertions. The Palmar interossei ADuct the fingers (PAD) and the Dorsal interossei ABduct the fingers (DAB). Figure 1.5 illustrates the lumbricles of the hand.

Nail bed injuries are common and you will be asked to deal with them on a daily basis, whether it is assessment or repair. It is therefore essential that you know the anatomy of this region well. Figure 1.6 illustrates an AP and lateral photography of a finger with superimposed diagrams of the anatomy. The nail is produced in the germinal matrix and grows distally.

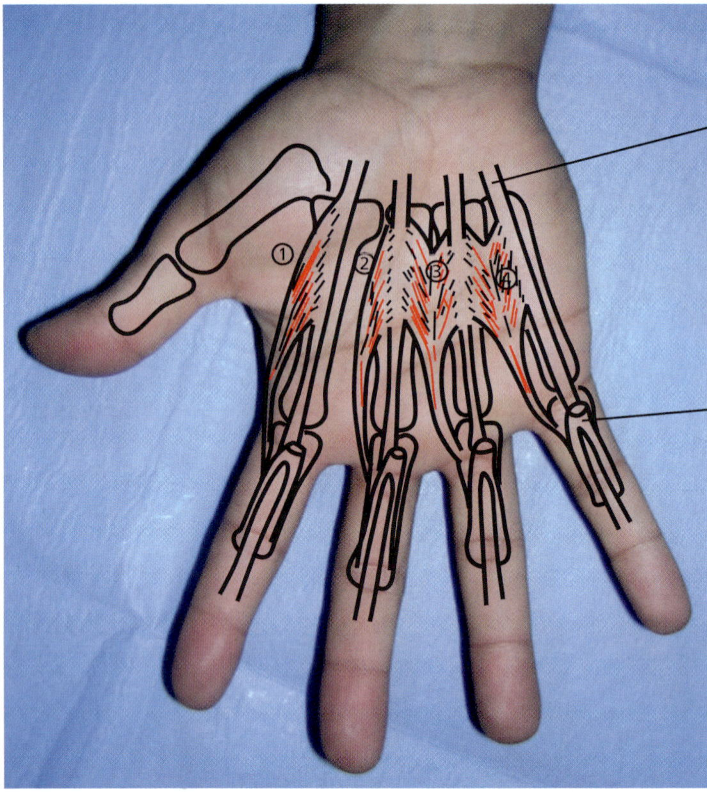


**Figure 1.5** Lumbricles

Power and sensation to the hand is supplied by three nerves that traverse the arm from their origin in the brachial plexus. Figures 1.8 and 1.9 illustrate the course and branches of these nerves. You should actively examine for sensory and motor deficit if injuries correlate with the anatomical course of these nerves. Finger injuries are common, so it is important to be familiar with the anatomy.

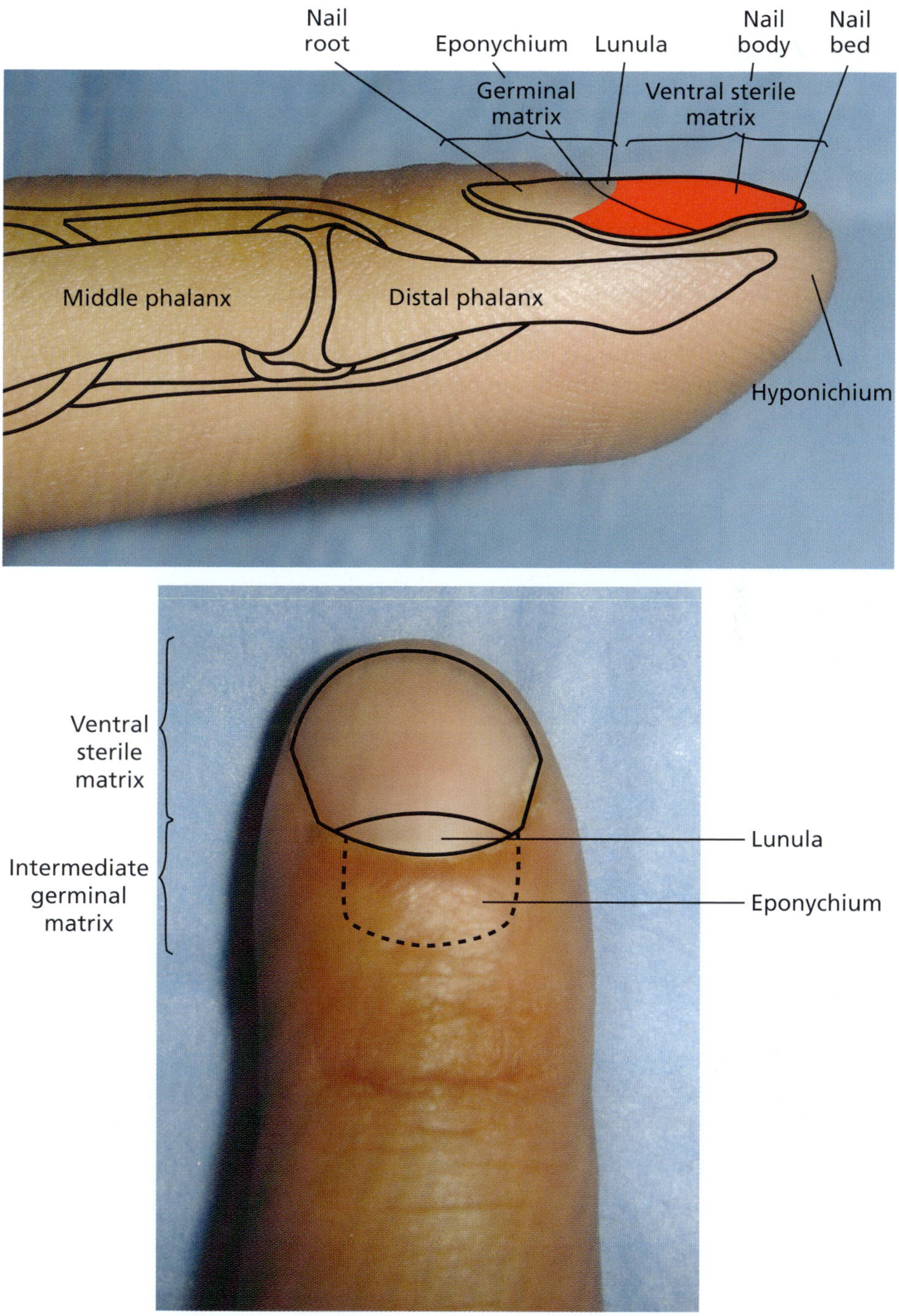


**Figure 1.6** Sagittal section of the fingertip of an index finger. Note that the neurovascular bundle runs on the palmar aspect of the finger

# History

Patients with severe injuries to the upper extremity should be checked routinely for accompanying injuries, which in some cases may be life threatening. About 10–15% of all patients with polytrauma have injuries to the hand or upper extremity.

It is important to acquire a patient's medical and social history, as decisions about the appropriate treatment are based on the factors shown in Table 1.5.

**Table 1.5** Factors that affect decisions about appropriate treatment.

| Factor | Comments |
|---|---|
| Age | |
| Occupation | • Technical skills<br>• Endurance<br>• Active range of movement<br>• Grip strength<br>• Sensitivity and coordination<br>• Socioeconomic issues (length of rehabilitation etc.)<br>• Psychological effects on patients (i.e. can the injured machinist return to the same machine) |
| Hand dominance | |
| Previous history of injury and outcome; and Previous surgery (to the hand), anaesthetic risk | |
| Mechanism of injury | • Crush – consider compartment syndrome, can cause severe cell damage making tissue viability less likely, look for fractures<br>• Contaminated – for debridement, early washout and surgery<br>• Blood loss – haemodynamic stability, active bleeding from a vessel<br>• Injury to underlying tendons<br>• Position of the hand at the time of injury - injury to underlying structures can mismatch the laceration site of the skin at the time of the examination |
| Time since injury – likely spread of contamination, degree of viability; and Place of injury<br>Environment<br>Last meal | • Clean or dirty, degree of contamination<br>• Last food six hours before surgery<br>• Last water two hours before surgery (other fluids are regarded in the food category) |
| Possible deliberate self-harm?<br>Degree of pain<br>Past medical history<br>Drug history<br>Allergies<br>Social history | • Early liaison with psychiatry and address of underlying problem<br>• Consider early regional anaesthesia for assessment*<br>• Including other and previous (hand) injuries<br>• Including tetanus immunization status<br>• Smoking – decreases perfusion in small vessels and delays healing of tendon, nerve and vessel repairs<br>• Alcohol – monitor mental state and look out for withdrawal symptoms. If patient is inebriated at referring hospital, then unless they need immediate surgery or treatment, admit the following day to avoid the problems drunk patients can cause on the ward |

*Digital nerve injuries are easy to miss in the first 24 hours – role your pen on the affected side of the finger and look for presence or absence of sweat which is a good sign of de-innervation.

# Examination

## Inspection

When examing a hand injury expose the *entire* limb and inspect carefully. It is important to illicit and record the following information.

- Site of injury
- Type of injury
  - Skin (loss, quality)
  - Nail bed
  - Laceration (linear or jagged)
  - Crush
  - Degloving
  - Clean/contaminated
  - Multiple injuries
  - Amputation (partial or complete)
  - Blood (active bleeding; arterial or venous)
  - Signs of previous scars (consider deliberate self-harm)
- Erythema and infection

Note that the patient may require analgesia and regional anaesthesia before undergoing further assessment.

## Palpation

Having carried out a thorough inspection, you should now palpate taking the below points into account during your examination to re-inforce your diagnosis.

- Temperature
- Surface irregularities, i.e. foreign bodies
- Oedema (which can limit movement)
- Moisture (nerve damage may cause the loss of ability to sweat)
- Muscles and their tendons
- Nerves
- Bone
- Ligaments

Always draw a diagram of the wound in the notes to give an idea of wound size, site and functional deficit. Consider arranging photographs for inclusion in the notes.

## Sensory assessment

Table 1.6 illustrates where to test for the sensory distribution of the various nerves supplying the hand. Figure 1.7 illustrates the sensory distribution of the three nerves supplying sensation to the hand. Note that there is crossover which in some cases may be significant.

**Table 1.6** Sensory assessment.

| Nerve | Location |
|---|---|
| Median nerve | • Pulp of thumb and index finger |
| Ulnar nerve | • Pulp of little finger and ulnar half of ring finger |
| Radial nerve | • Dorsal first web space |
| Palmar cutaneous nerve | • Proximal thenar eminence |
| Dorsal cutaneous branch of the ulnar nerve | • Dorsal ulnar aspect of hand |

## Motor assessment

Table 1.7 demonstrates intrinsic and extrinsic motor innervation of the muscles of the hand by the radial, ulnar and median nerves.

**Table 1.7** Motor assessment.

| Nerve | Location |
|---|---|
| Median nerve | |
| Intrinsic | • Thumb palmar abduction |
| Extrinsic | • All flexor digitorum superficialis<br>• Flexor pollicus longus<br>• Flexor digitorum profundus to index finger<br>• Flexor carpi radialis |
| Ulnar nerve | |
| Intrinsic | • Dorsal interossei muscles<br>• Abduction/adduction: hypothenar muscles |
| Extrinsic | • Flexor digitorum profundus to little finger<br>• Flexor carpi ulnaris |
| Radial nerve | |
| Extrinsic | • Extension of wrist<br>• Extension of thumb<br>• Extension of MP joints |

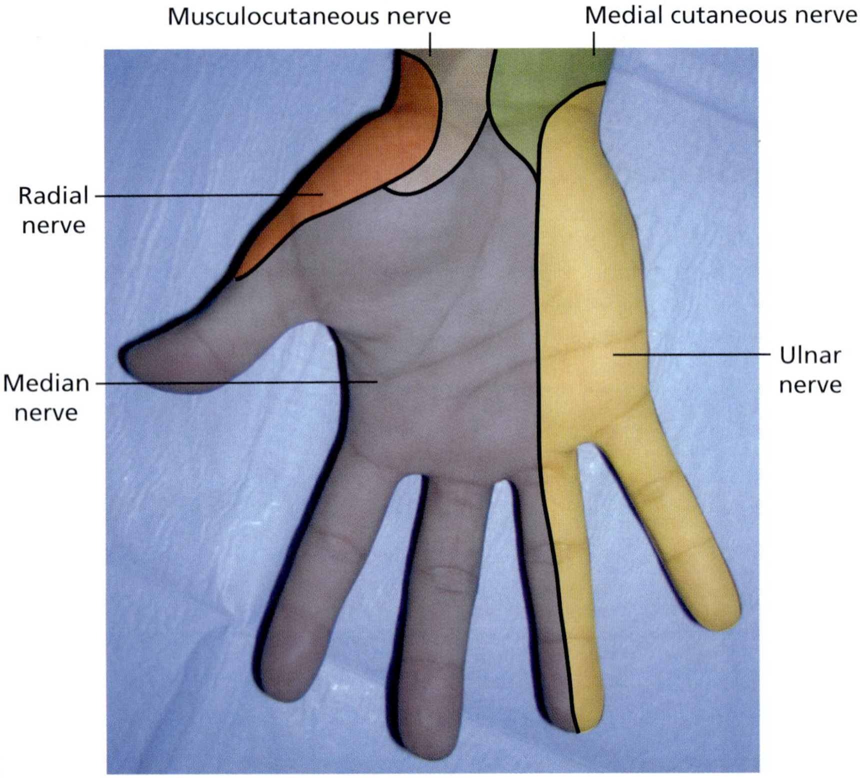


(a)

**Figure 1.7** Distribution of sensory nerves in the hand and their territory of innervation: (a) palmar view (*continued*)

## Treatment goals

The goals of treatment are:

- preservation and restoration of function
- salvage of extremities
- analgesia
- correction of acquired defects
- optimal aesthetic appearance
- social and professional reintegration
- cost-effective therapy.

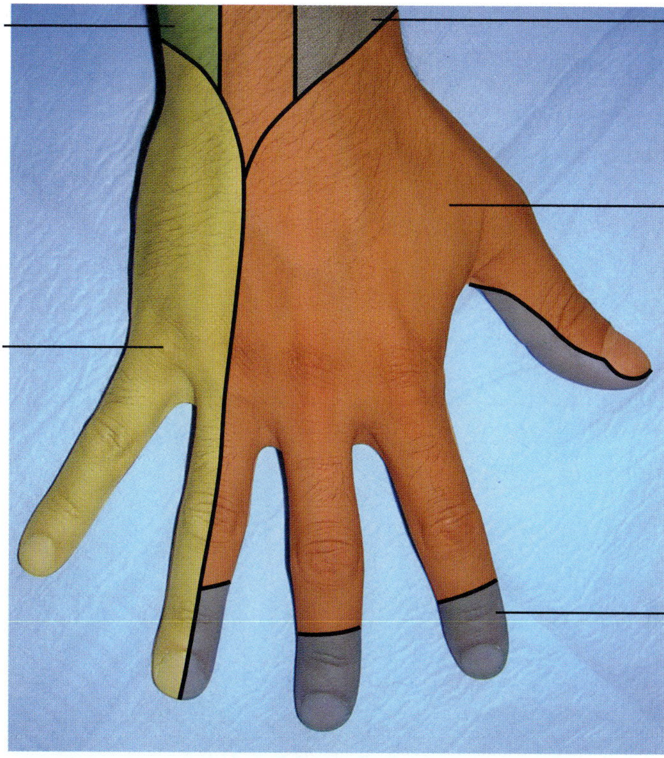


(b)

**Figure 1.7** (*continuted*) Distribution of sensory nerves in the hand and their territory of innervation: (b) dorsal view

Figures 1.8 and 1.9 illustrate the course of the various nerves and vessels traversing the arm, superimposed on a photograph to allow you to orientate yourself. Familiarize yourself with these as you will need to test for their function where injuries correspond to their cause.

Figures 1.10–1.13 illustrate how to perform various tests in your clinical examination. Figure 1.10 shows how to test finger abduction which is a test of the ulnar nerve. Figure 1.11 illustrates testing thumb abduction which is a test of the median nerve. Figures 1.12 and 1.13 show a good way of testing the flexor digitorum profundus (FDP) and flexor digitorum superficialis (FDS) tendons.

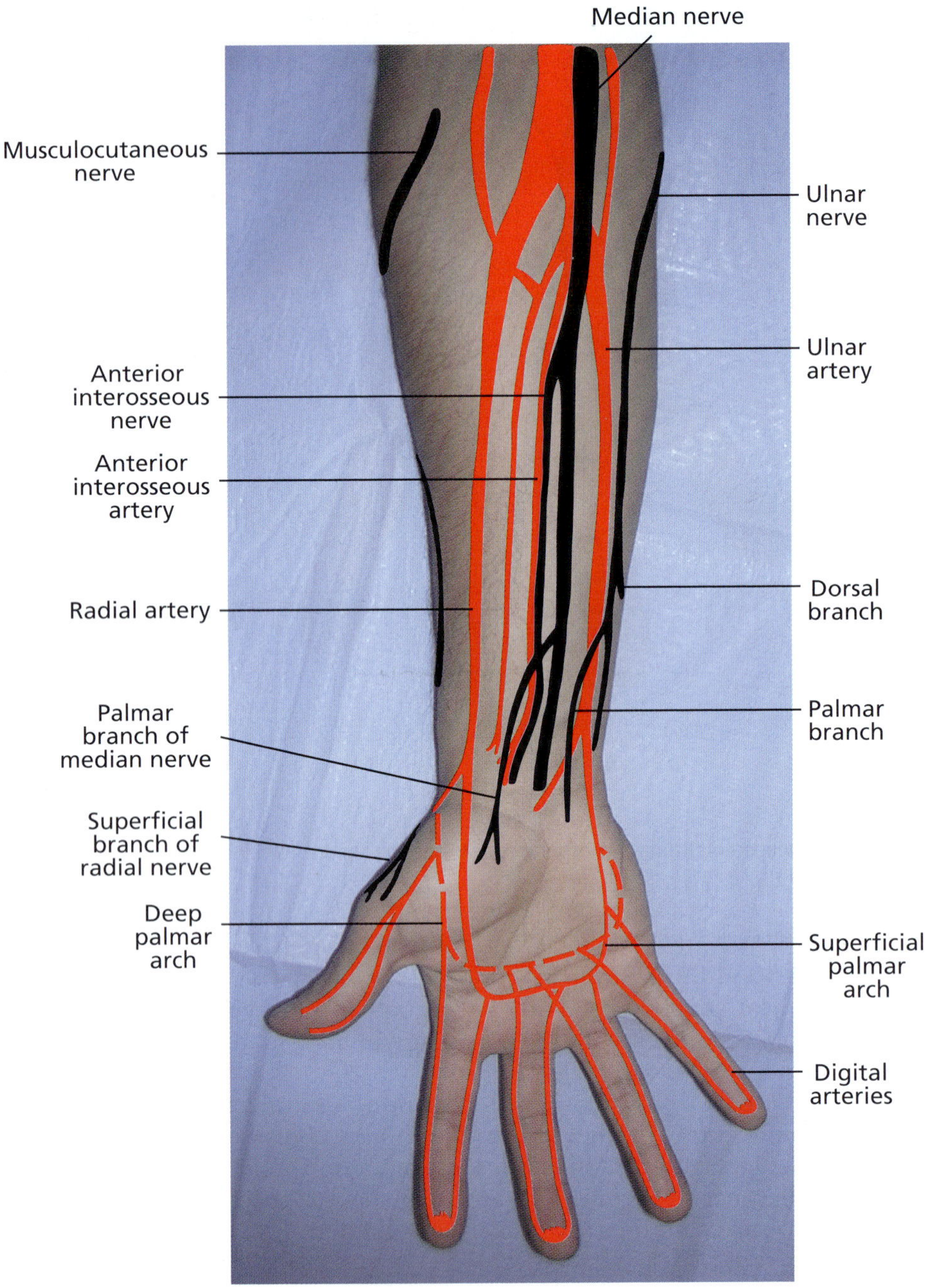


**Figure 1.8** Course of the nerves and vessels of the forearm

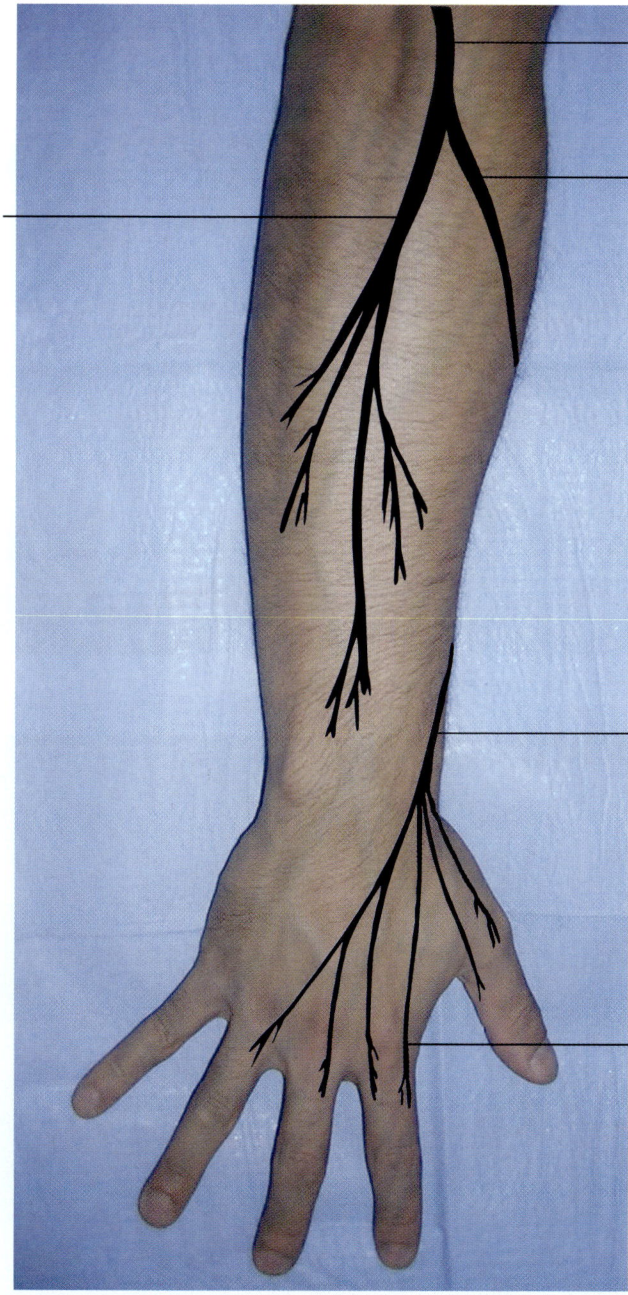


**Figure 1.9** Course of the radial nerve in the forearm

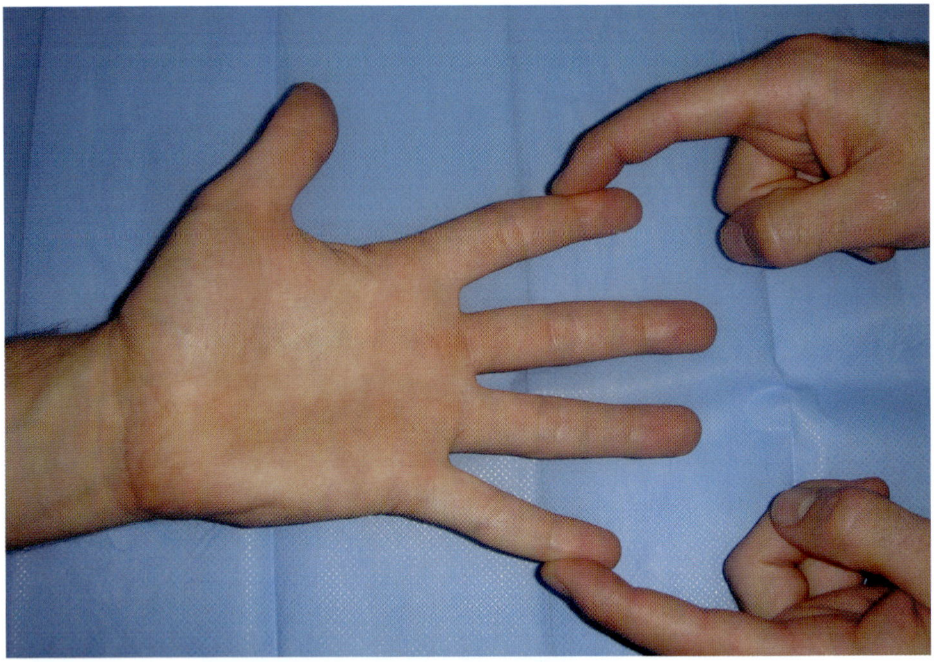

**Figure 1.10** Testing finger abduction

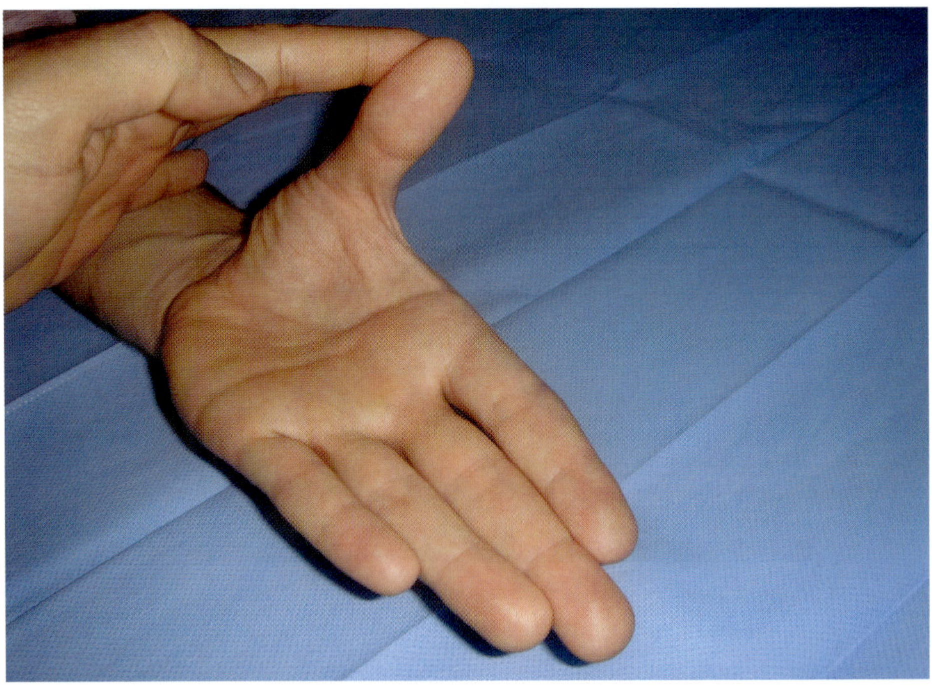

**Figure 1.11** Testing thumb abduction

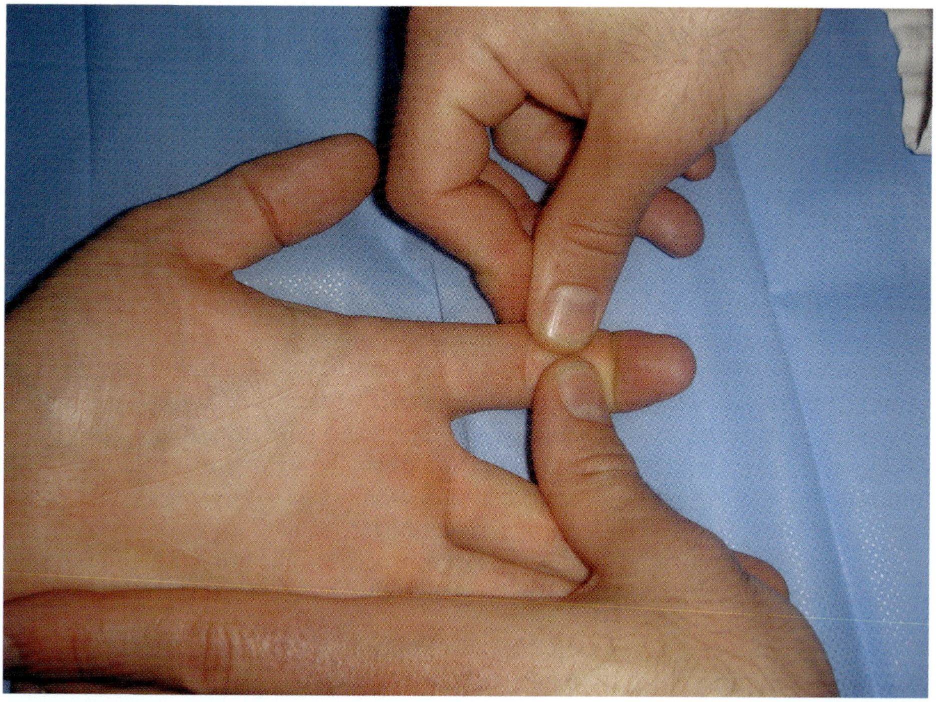

**Figure 1.12** Testing the flexor digitorum profundus

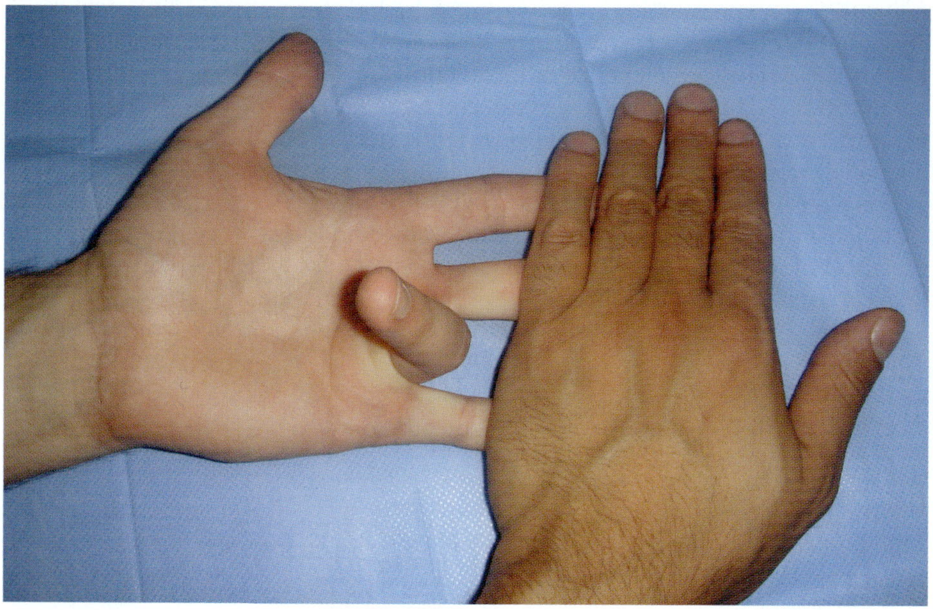

**Figure 1.13** Testing the flexor digitorum superficialis

# Local anaesthetic blocks

You may need to administer a local anaesthetic (LA) during elective and trauma lists, during minor operations lists and when suturing in the emergency department. Local anaesthetics can be infiltrated locally or given as a regional (e.g. axillary) or nerve (e.g. median) block.

It can be very helpful to combine LA with added adrenaline – usually at a ratio of 1:80,000 – as this significantly reduces bleeding from the wound edges; however, local anaesthesia should *not* be combined with adrenaline in the case of digital block, penile block or a laceration of the hand. It is a good idea to use a mixture of a short-acting LA and a longer acting LA: for example, 5 ml of 1% lignocaine plus 5 ml of 0.25% bupivacaine (marcaine) will give you the benefits of fast onset (lignocaine) and long duration (bupivacaine). The maximum doses of local anaesthetic are:

- 3 mg/kg lidocaine (7 mg/kg with adrenaline)
- 2 mg/kg bupivacaine (alone or with adrenaline).

The LA should be injected slowly and preferably warmed to room temperature to reduce the pain of injection. You should use the smallest needle possible. Tell the patient to expect a stinging sensation, which is due to the acidity of the local anaesthetic solution. When injecting, keep the needle moving and inject as you withdraw to reduce the chance of intravenous or intra-arterial injection. If you are injecting in the region of a nerve and the patient experiences sudden, shooting and very unpleasant pain, withdraw the needle because you are probably injecting into the nerve.

The effects of LA and adrenaline are not instantaneous, so you should wait for at least five minutes after local infiltration – and longer for digital and nerve blocks – before you begin any surgery. A ring block for anaesthetizing the pinna takes at least 20 minutes to work.

Beware of the risk of systemic toxicity if LA is injected into a vessel. Symptoms include:

- perioral tingling
- tinnitus
- confusion
- fitting
- loss of consciousness
- cardiac arrhythmia
- cardiac arrest.

If any of these symptoms occur, treat the symptoms; check the airway, breathing and circulation (ABC) and call for help.

## Local infiltration

Local infiltration into the dermis of the edges of a wound is particularly useful for anaesthetizing superficial skin lacerations that do not need extending or much exploration. You will frequently be asked to suture facial lacerations, which are discussed in the section on facial trauma (page 103). Inject the anaesthetic into the dermis, where the nociceptive nerve plexi are located, rather than the subcutaneous fat. In patients with lacerations, inject the LA a few millimetres from the wound edges so that you do not distort the edges and make suturing inaccurate.

### *Digital blocks*

Digital blocks are useful for repairs of the nail bed, digital nerve and extensor tendon. They entail blocking the ulnar and radial digital nerves at the base of the digit (Figure 1.14).

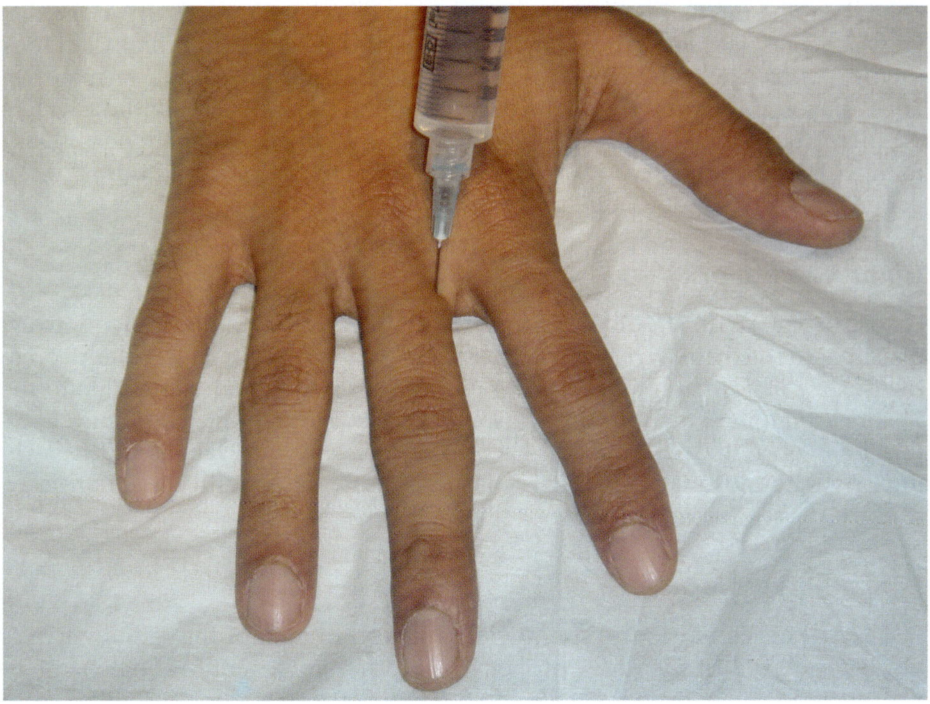

**Figure 1.14** Administering a digital block

Use a 50:50 mixture of lidocaine and bupivacaine *without adrenaline*. A dose of 8 ml should suffice for one digit. Inject dorsally into the webspace on either side of the digit. Dorsal injections are less painful because the skin is not bound down to fascia and thus allows swelling. For the thumb radial digital nerve and little finger ulnar digital nerves, simply infiltrate at the same level at which you inject the LA on the other side of the digit. The fingertip may take as long as 20 minutes to become anaesthetized but it is usually numb within a few minutes.

## Wrist blocks

The purpose of a wrist block is to anaesthetize part or all of the hand. A wrist block can block a single nerve or all of the nerves that supply the hand (regional block). The nerves that enter the hand through the wrist are the radial, median and ulnar nerves. The nerve you block depends on the part of the hand on which you wish to operate (see Figure 1.7). Different techniques can be used to block these nerves. The correct technique is the technique that works for you. The techniques described below are the authors' preferences.

### *Median nerve block*

A dose of 10 ml of LA should be more than enough. Approach the carpal tunnel, where the median nerve runs, by inserting the needle vertically at the distal wrist crease between the palmaris longus and flexor carpi radialis tendons (Figure 1.15). Angle the needle volarly after piercing the skin. You may feel 'give' as you pass through the flexor retinaculum. Inject as you withdraw. It is useful to raise a bleb distally to block the palmar cutaneous branch. As it is easy to inject the median nerve itself, keep the needle moving and withdraw if the patient gets any sudden pain.

### *Ulnar nerve block*

A dose of 5 ml of LA should be enough. Find the flexor carpi ulnaris tendon just proximal to the distal wrist crease. Pass the needle from dorsal to volar deep to the flexor carpi ulnaris tendon and raise a bleb on the volar skin radial to the flexor carpi ulnaris tendon (this shows you are in the right place) (Figure 1.16). Inject as you withdraw and raise a bleb on the way out. This is particularly important, because the ulnar artery is closely associated with the ulnar nerve (the artery is radial to the nerve).

### *Radial nerve block*

In a radial nerve block, the superficial (sensory) branch of the radial nerve is blocked rather than the nerve proper. The block involves infiltrating 5–7 ml of LA subcutaneously from just radial to the radial artery at the wrist and continuing dorsally to the midpoint of the wrist (Figure 1.17).

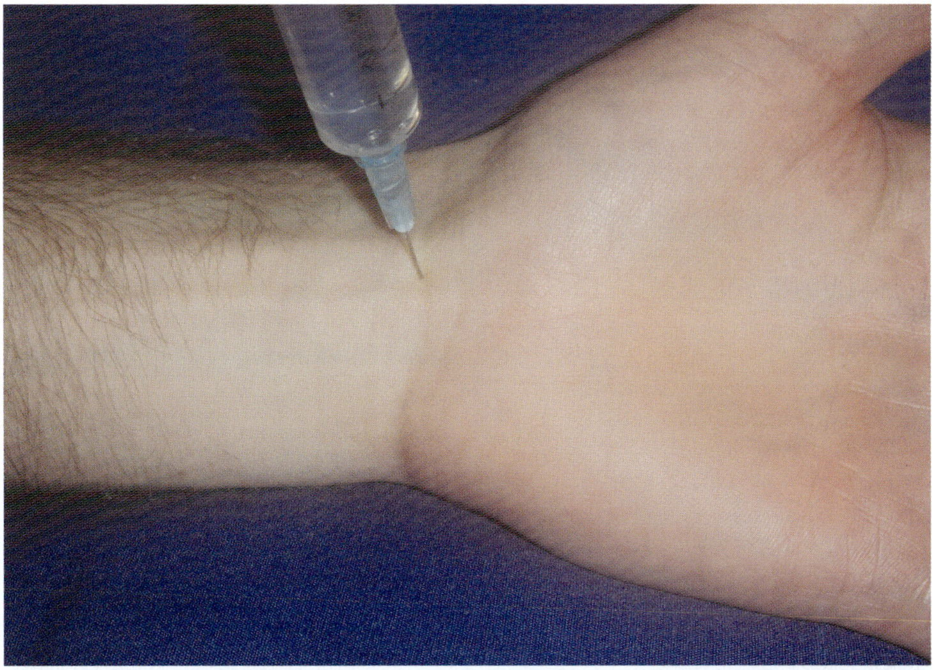

**Figure 1.15** Administering a median nerve block

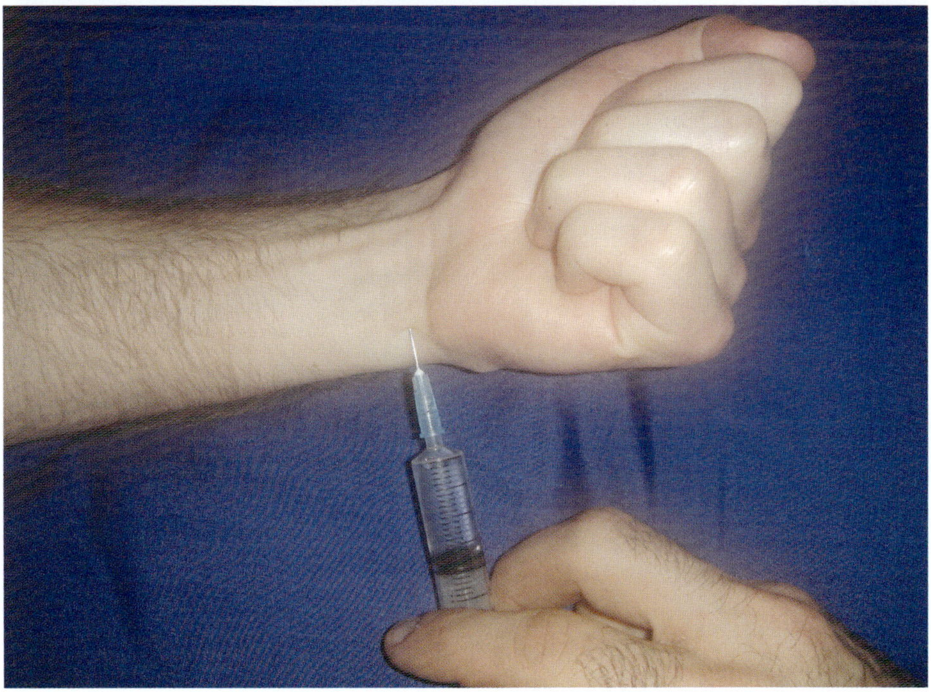

**Figure 1.16** Administering an ulnar nerve block

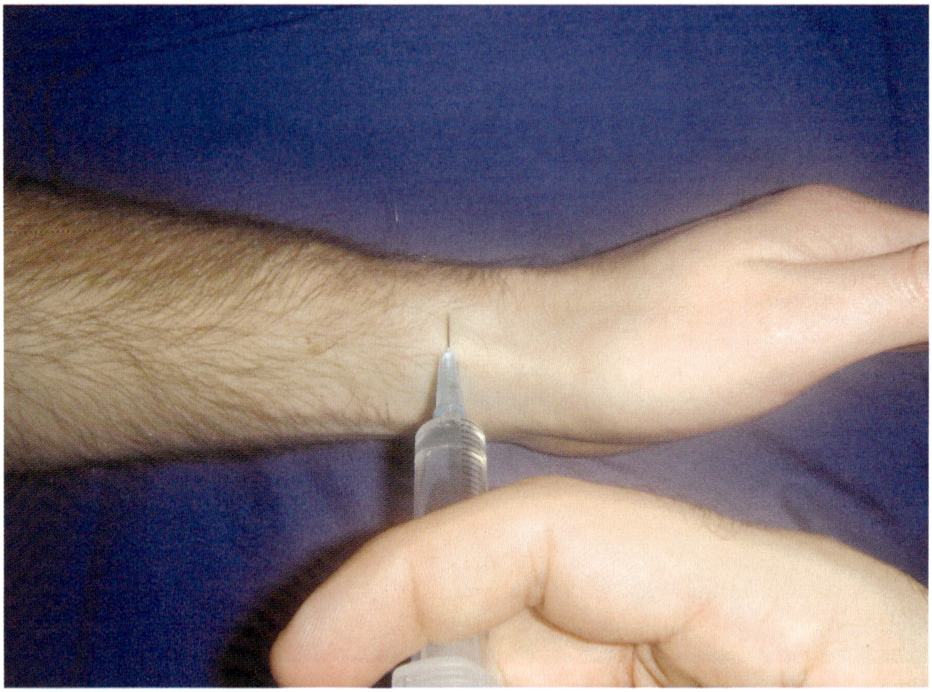

**Figure 1.17** Administering a radial nerve block

# Nail-bed injuries

Fingernails protect fingertips from trauma, aid fine grip and prevent deformation of digital skin, which contributes to the sensitivity of the fingertip demonstrated by the two-point discrimination test.

Nail-bed injuries are the most common type of hand injury, particularly in children. They are usually caused by crush mechanisms, particularly when the fingertip is caught in a closing door. The nail bed is deep to the nail and extends proximally deep to the eponychium as the germinal matrix (see Figures 1.6 and 1.18). Destruction of the germinal matrix usually results in permanent loss of the fingernail. A subungal haematoma is caused by a laceration of the nail bed and so should be treated in the same way as a nail-bed injury despite the nail itself being intact. A painful haematoma can be relieved by piercing the overlying nail with a needle. Nail-bed injuries are often associated with fracture of the distal phalanx, so make sure to ask the referring doctor to send radiographs with the patient.

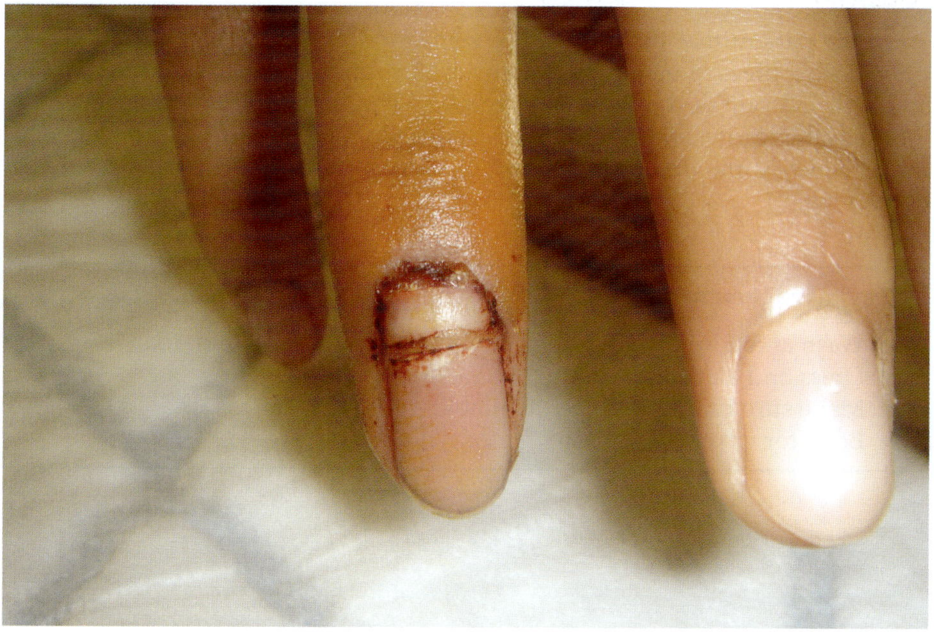

**Figure 1.18** An avulsed finger nail – the nail will need to be removed, any associated nail-bed laceration repaired and then the nail reinserted under the nail fold to splint it open until a new nail grows.

Patients with nail-bed injuries do not have to be admitted or operated on immediately and can safely wait until the next trauma list unless there is any suspicion that the vascular supply of the distal finger is compromised. Advise the referring doctor to give the patient a course of oral antibiotics in the interim and to irrigate the wound, especially if it is contaminated or there is an underlying fracture (which is therefore an open fracture). Ask the doctor to check the patient's tetanus vaccination status and to vaccinate if required. Remember to confirm the tetanus status with the patient once they are admitted.

Nail-bed injuries in adults can be repaired under LA. In injuries associated with fractures of the underlying terminal phalanx, the surgeon may choose to stabilize the fracture with a K-wire. Although this can be performed under LA, many surgeons prefer a general anaesthetic (GA) for this procedure, so keep this in mind when preparing the patient.

The aim of treatment is to preserve function and prevent deformity or loss of the nail. Surgical management of nail-bed injuries includes:

- assessment of the underlying nail-bed injury by removing the nail
- stabilization of the distal phalanx, if required
- repair of the nail bed and any associated skin laceration
- replacement of the missing sterile matrix with sterile matrix graft as the primary procedure
- replacement of the nail plate to act as a splint.

Warn the patient that the nail will be reinserted under the nail fold or substituted with a piece of metal foil. These act as temporary splints for the nail fold and will fall out as the new nail regrows. The new nail will take up to six months to regrow and, because of underlying damage to the nail bed, it may display some deformity, although surgery decreases the chance of that happening.

**Key management points**

- Wash and administer antibiotics if the injury is contaminated
- Dress and elevate the hand
- Make sure radiographs are available
- Book for next LA list

# Mallet finger

Mallet fingers are (closed) avulsion injuries of the zone I extensor tendon and are caused by sudden forced flexion of the distal interphalangeal joint, such as a football hitting the end of the finger. Most can be treated conservatively with eight weeks' continuous splinting followed by two weeks' splinting at night only, although the exact protocol will vary from unit to unit. Patients can be discharged in a mallet splint and brought back to the hand clinic in 1–2 weeks.

If an underlying avulsion fracture of the terminal phalanx is present, the patient *may* need surgery. If the patient has an open mallet injury, the patient *will* need surgery.

In the case of avulsion fractures, the need for surgery depends on the size of the fragment, the extent of intra-articular involvement and the presence of unacceptable volar subluxation of the distal phalanx. Surgery usually involves passing one or two K-wires across the distal interphalangeal joint. Roughly speaking, fragments that involve more than one quarter of the joint surface or that are >4 mm across may need surgery, so discuss the radiographs with your registrar. In patients with smaller fragments, splint as previously and arrange a hand clinic appointment about a week later.

Open mallet injuries need surgery because the joint space is likely to be breached due to the superficiality of the joint and extensor tendons. Patients with open mallet injuries should receive oral antibiotics (or intravenous antibiotics if the wound is contaminated) and be listed for washout of the joint on a list within the next 24 hours. When obtaining the patient's consent, you should explain that the surgeon may insert a K-wire across the joint in place of a mallet splint.

**Key management points**

- Closed mallet injuries with or without small avulsion fragments: treat with mallet splint
- Patients with large avulsion fragments or intra-articular involvement: may need surgery under LA
- Open mallet injuries: oral antibiotics and washout of joints under LA

# Nerve injuries

Most nerve injuries that you will be referred will involve the hand, but you should always consider and examine for nerve injuries in patients with trauma to other parts of the body. Nerve injuries are usually caused by lacerations and are noticed by the patient as a change in sensation or, rarely as a loss of movement. Neither the patient nor the referring person may necessarily detect any change in sensation or movement, however, do not assume a nerve is undamaged in the absence of symptoms or signs. All wounds in the upper limb that breach, or may breach, the dermis should be explored for occult involvement of nerves, vessels, muscles, tendons and joints.

The most common nerve injury you will see is a digital nerve injury. Patients with these injuries should ideally be admitted for the next available trauma list, but they could wait for several days as long as the injury has been washed out, no other injuries are present and they are given cover with oral antibiotics. Remember that the digital nerves run with the digital arteries, so injury to one usually also means injury to the other. When a digital nerve injury is referred, therefore, specifically ask the referring doctor about perfusion of the finger. If both radial and ulnar digital nerves are damaged, see the patient straight away, as the finger may need to be revascularized. Single digital nerve injuries can be repaired under LA with a finger tourniquet, but more complicated injuries may need a GA.

Injuries of the median, ulnar and, less frequently, radial and superficial radial nerves will also be referred. Patients with such injuries should ideally be seen straight away, because damage to these nerves, particularly the median and ulnar nerves, raises the possibility of damage to the major arteries to the hand and because they are likely to be complicated injuries that will benefit from prompt elevation, pain control, possible intravenous antibiotics and early surgery. If you are sure there is no concomitant arterial injury, however, the patient could be seen the next day. These injuries, except potentially isolated superficial radial nerve injuries, will need to be explored under GA.

When obtaining consent from patients, remember that the point of nerve repair is to restore continuity of the nerve to prevent formation of painful neuromas. This also gives the best chance of the nerve recovering its function, but recovery may be only partial, especially in the case of injuries of the major nerves. After surgery, the patient will likely have a splint and require several months of physiotherapy in the case of injury to the major nerves. Nerve recovery takes about 18 months. You should also warn patients that they will need a nerve graft if primary repair is impossible. This would usually be a cutaneous sensory nerve taken from the forearm and would, of course, mean one or two more scars and an area of paraesthesia over the forearm that should slowly improve over 18 months or more.

**Key management points**

- Consider vascular involvement
- Elevate the arm and administer oral antibiotics
- Isolated digital nerve injuries: repair under LA within one week
- Injuries of median, ulnar and radial nerves: repair under GA on the next trauma list

# Tendon injuries

Tendon injuries are very common and you will see many of them. They may be present even if you see no functional deficit on examination, because tendon divisions may be incomplete and many hand movements are accomplished by more than one muscle. It is generally best to assume that a patient has a tendon injury if a laceration is found over a tendon and especially if the cause was something sharp, such as glass.

Your colleagues will often describe tendon injuries in terms of zones, which are useful because they describe the location of the injury but also indicate the surgery that will be needed to repair the tendon and the likely prognosis. Generally speaking, the more distal the laceration, the harder it is to repair and the worse the prognosis.

Figure 1.19 illustrates the various flexor and extensor zones in the hand. These zones should be used to describe injuries. Remember that the extensor zones are numbered such that odd numbers are over joints – i.e. zone I over distal interphalangeal joint, zone III over proximal interphalangeal joint, etc.

Admit patients with tendon injuries, give oral antibiotics (intravenous antibiotics in the case of contaminated wounds) and elevate the limb in a Bradford sling. If there is no vascular compromise, immediate admission is not imperative, although the injury ideally should be repaired within 24 hours.

Remember that tendons become increasingly difficult to repair primarily (i.e. joining the ends directly together) as time progresses, because the proximal tendon retracts as the muscle contracts. Two weeks is probably the absolute cut-off point for injuries of the flexor tendons, after which repair is possible only with tendon grafts or transfers. As a general guide, if you cannot arrange surgery for a patient with a flexor tendon injury within five days of injury , then rather than accept the referral suggest that the patient is referred to another unit.

## Palm lacerations

Palm lacerations are included here, as deep palm lacerations will often involve the flexor tendons. It is worth remembering that the digital arteries arise from the superficial palmar arch, which is *superficial* to the flexor tendons. A patient with a palm laceration and a flexor tendon deficit should be seen promptly, as the involved digits may need revascularizing.

Lacerations of the extensor tendons, unless multiple, can usually be repaired under LA, because they are superficial and do not tend to retract because of the

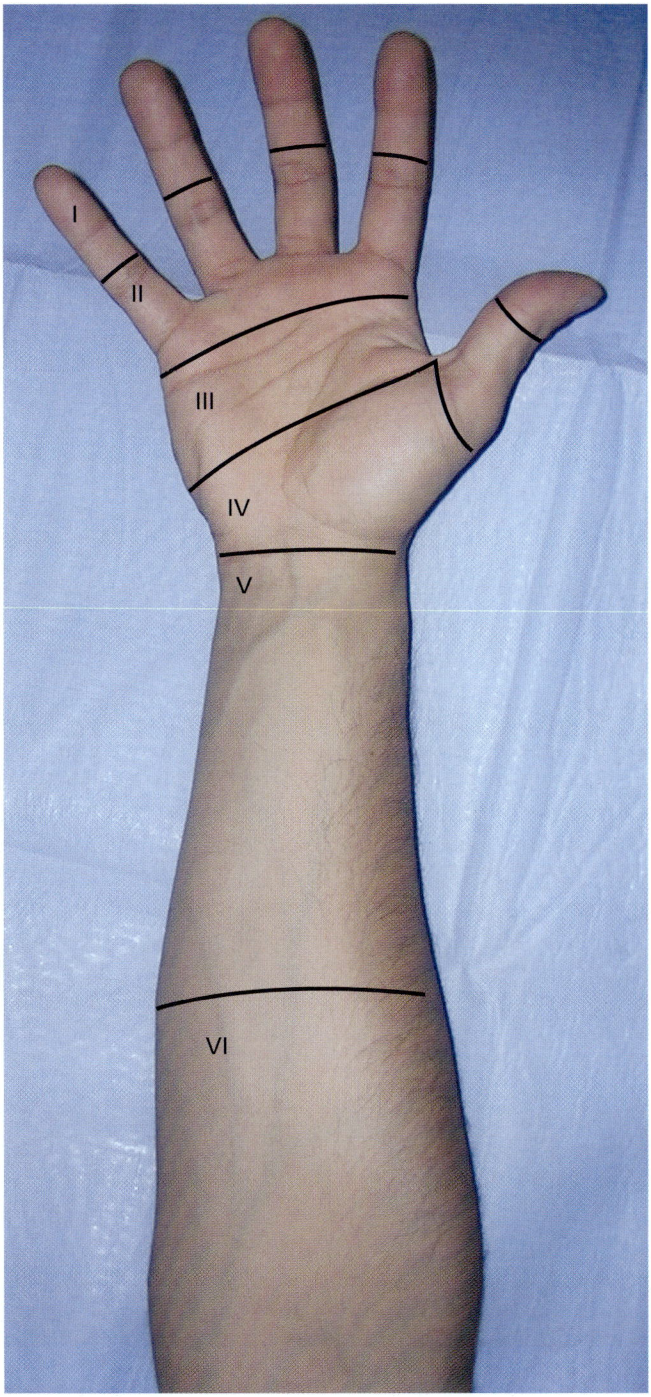


(a)

**Figure 1.19** (a) The zones of flexor tendon injury (*continued*)

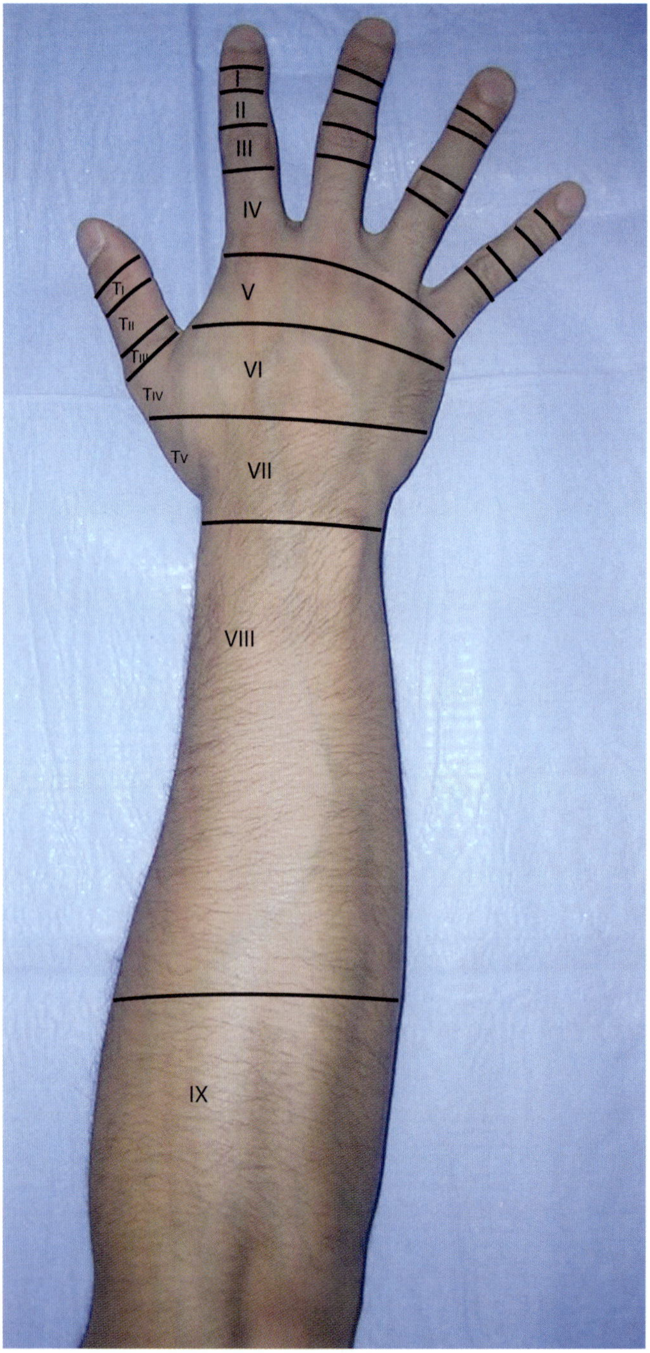


(b)

**Figure 1.19** (*continued*) (b) The zones of extensor tendon injury

junctura tendinae. They are also relatively quick to repair: the arm tourniquet does not need to be inflated for more than 25 minutes and the surgery can be completed before the discomfort from the tourniquet becomes unbearable. On the other hand, lacerations of the flexor tendons tend to take longer to repair, because the tendons are deeper, damage to other structures is more likely and the tendons retract because there are no junctura tendinae. All flexor lacerations should be booked for repair under GA. These guidelines also apply to injuries of thumb tendons, although many registrars prefer to repair thumb extensors with the patient under GA too.

As with all injuries, look out for vascular compromise. This is more likely with flexor injuries, because most of the neurovascular structures are volar.

When obtaining consent, tell the patient that they will have a splint after their operation, they will need physiotherapy and they will not be able to use their hand fully for up to three months. For many people, this will mean being off work for this time. Warn patients not to smoke, as this will impair healing of the tendons.

**Key management points**

- Dress, elevate and administer oral antibiotics
- Flexor injuries: admit, repair under GA within five days of injury
- Extensor injuries: repair usually under LA

# Hand fractures

Hand fractures are common and most can be treated conservatively. Important findings are fractures that interfere with function because of angulation or rotation, intra-articular fractures, open fractures and inherently unstable fractures. These will need surgery, and you should admit patients with these injuries or at least discuss them with your registrar.

As with all hand injuries, elevation is vital. Most closed, stable fractures require very little immobilization except for pain control, and immediate mobilization within the limits of comfort is ideal to prevent long-term stiffness. Phalangeal fractures can be simply buddy-strapped. Metacarpal fractures, unless multiple, are already splinted by the other metacarpals in the hand. Carpal fractures require a backslab only to control pain.

Patients with open fractures of the hand should be given antibiotics, which should be given orally in the case of uncontaminated terminal phalanx fractures. Patients with all other fractures should receive intravenous antibiotics to avoid osteomyelitis and septic arthritis, which are difficult to treat and disastrous for the patient.

Patients with fractures that meet the criteria for conservative treatment (closed, stable, no deformity, pain under control) can be discharged home. They should be given instructions to mobilize the hand within the limits of pain and without force. The patient should be given an appointment for hand therapy the same week to minimize the delay if the position of the fracture changes or surgery becomes warranted. If there is any suspicion of a change in position of the fracture, radiographs should be taken in the first two weeks. After two weeks, healing of the fracture makes reduction and surgery increasingly difficult.

If a patient's fracture falls outside the above criteria, or you are unsure, do not discharge the patient without at least showing the radiographs to your registrar. Do not worry about admitting a patient overnight in anticipation of surgery and your registrar later deciding to pursue conservative treatment: the patient will still have benefited from the elevation and pain control.

## Fractures of the terminal phalanx (fingers and thumb)

Fractures of the terminal (distal) phalanx are often accompanied by nail-bed injuries and, in such cases, constitute open fractures (Figure 1.20). Patients with such injuries should be treated with oral antibiotics and admitted for the next trauma list for irrigation, nail-bed repair and usually K-wire fixation of the fracture under LA.

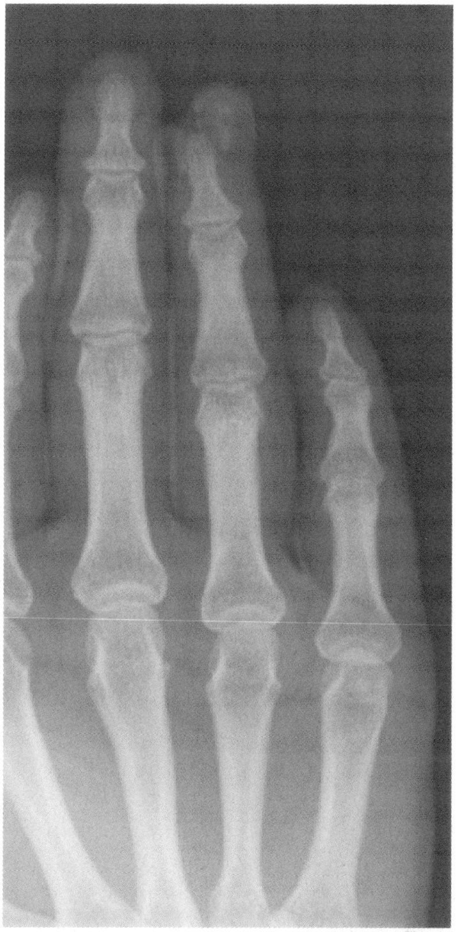

(a)

**Figure 1.20** Distal phalanx fractures: (a) tuft fracture (*continued*)

Closed fractures of the tuft or stable minimally deformed fractures of the distal shaft can be treated conservatively with a mallet splint for protection and pain control. Arrange a hand clinic appointment within a week.

Most proximal fractures are treated essentially as mallet fractures (see page 35). Other proximal fractures may need fixation with a K-wire because of the destabilizing effect of the tendon insertions in the proximal part of the phalanx. Review these patients with your registrar.

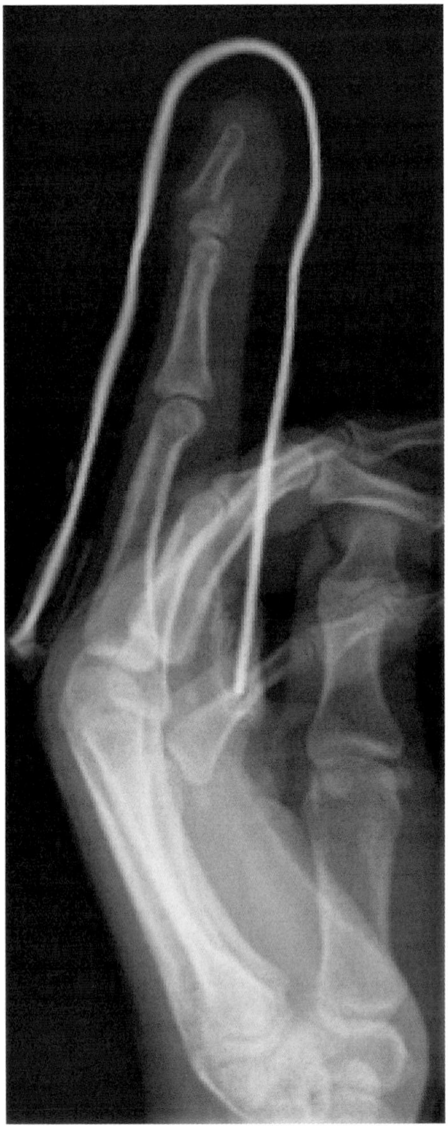

(b)

**Figure 1.20** (*continued*) Distal phalanx fractures: (b) fracture of the bone

**Key management points**

- Closed tuft fractures: mallet splint, review in hand clinic in one week
- Closed proximal fractures: treat as mallet injuries, may need K-wire fixation under LA
- Open fractures: oral antibiotics, book on next trauma list for irrigation (with or without K-wire fixation) under LA

## Fractures of the proximal and middle phalanges

Closed, undisplaced, minimally angulated transverse or oblique fractures of the proximal and middle phalanges (Figures 1.21 and 1.22) can be treated conservatively with buddy strapping. The patient should be sent home with an appointment for the hand clinic (with radiographs to be taken on arrival) in one week and instructions to mobilize within the limits of pain and elevate on pillows when at rest.

If a potentially stable fracture is in an unsatisfactory position – angulation of more than 10° in any direction or clinically rotated – consider reducing the fracture in the emergency department after administering a ring block (Figures 1.21 and 1.22). In practice, except in the case of joint dislocations, reduction of phalangeal fractures outside the operating theatre is rarely necessary or appropriate, and you should discuss these cases with your registrar before attempting any reduction. If you do attempt reduction and it is successful (confirm this with radiographs), buddy strap and bring the patient back to the clinic in one week. If reduction is unsuccessful, admit for surgery under GA the following day.

Fractures that are displaced with less than 50% bony contact, are angulated more than 10° or are off-ended, spiral, oblique or severely comminuted are unstable (Figure 1.23). Fractures of the neck of the proximal phalanx also should be considered unstable. Patients with these fractures should be admitted, as surgery under GA will be necessary.

If the finger is visibly deformed or neurovascularly compromised, it may be necessary to reduce immediately in the emergency department or in theatre, where definitive surgery can be carried out. Clearly, patients with such injuries should be reviewed urgently with your registrar.

Intra-articular fractures can be splinted if completely undisplaced, but the patient should be seen in clinic within a week or sooner. Patients with displaced intra-articular fractures should be admitted for surgery the next day under GA. Patients with displaced avulsion fractures at the bases of the proximal phalanges, particularly of the index and little fingers or thumb, also should be admitted for surgery.

Dislocations of the interphalangeal joints should be reduced as soon as possible to prevent neurovascular compromise. This can be achieved using a digital block and traction followed by buddy strapping and elevation. If this proves impossible, reduction under GA is required urgently. Review all

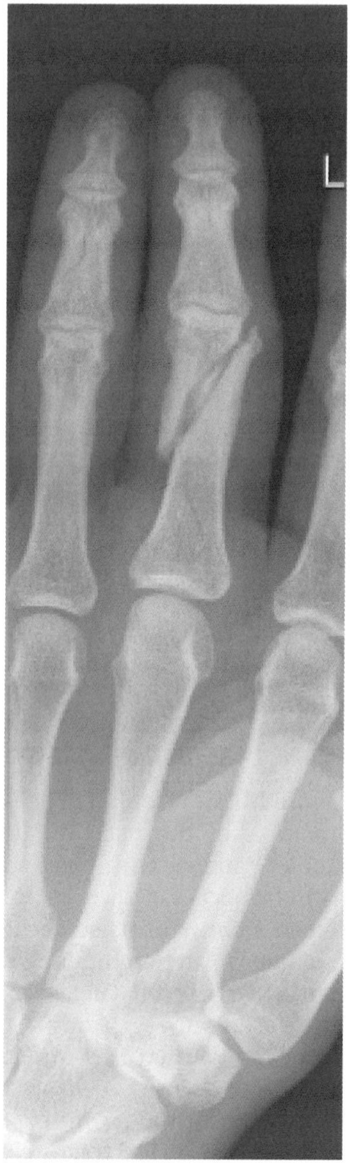


**Figure 1.21** An oblique fracture of the proximal phalanx. This fracture is displaced and unstable. It needs reduction and fixation (percutaneous, internal or external)

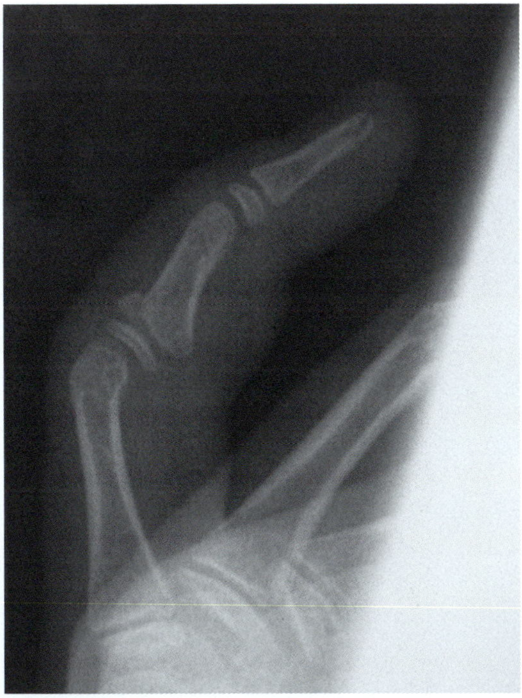

**Figure 1.22** A (Salter Harris II) fracture of the base of the middle phalanx

dislocations with your registrar, as stabilizing surgery may be required, especially if there is marked joint instability.

Patients with open fractures of the phalanges should be admitted for surgery – ideally within 24 hours but earlier if contaminated. These fractures should also be irrigated under ring block in the emergency department. Intravenous antibiotics are mandatory.

**Key management points**

- Closed, undisplaced, stable fractures: conservative treatment, mobilization, review in hand clinic in one week
- Closed unstable fractures: admit for reduction and fixation under GA
- Open fractures: admit; intravenous antibiotics; irrigation, reduction and fixation under GA within 24 hours
- Dislocations: reduce immediately under ring block, admit for possible exploration and stabilization under GA

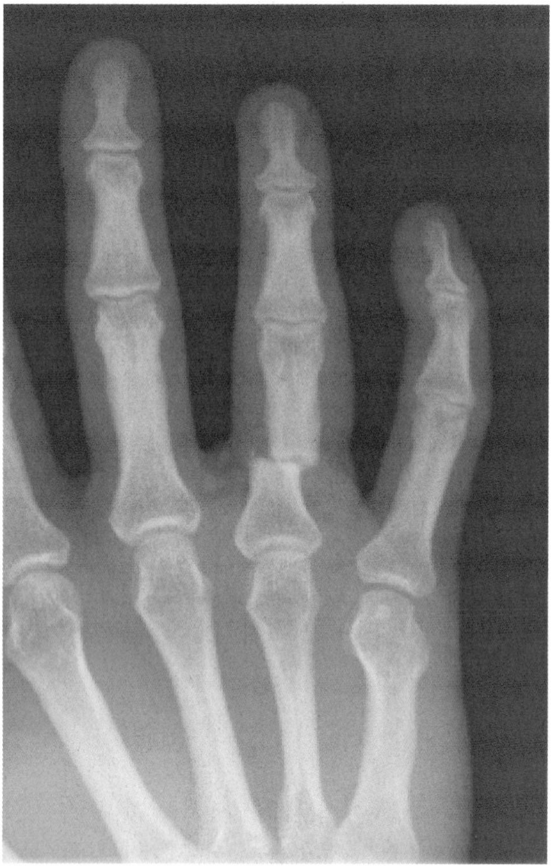

(a)

**Figure 1.23** Proximal phalanx fractures: (a) displaced transverse fracture of the proximal phalanx (*continued*)

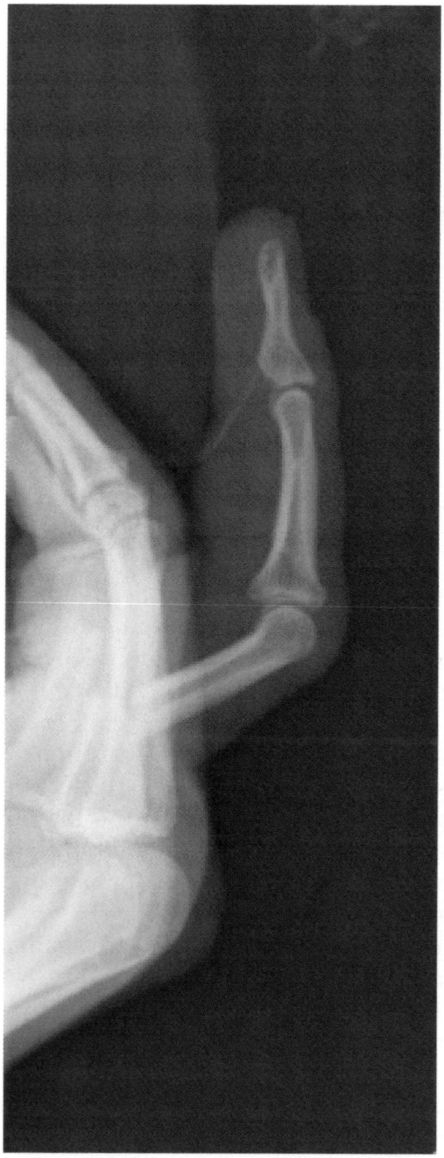

(b)

**Figure 1.23** (*continued*) Proximal phalanx fractures: (b) a dorsally angulated fracture of the proximal shaft of the proximal phalanx. This fracture needs immediate reduction to prevent ischaemia of the finger

## Fractures of the metacarpals

Isolated undisplaced, minimally angulated, non-rotated closed metacarpal fractures can be treated conservatively. A backslab may be required for pain control. Elevation is essential, as swelling can be severe. Look carefully for rotation. The patient should be seen in the hand clinic (with radiographs taken on arrival) within one week.

Patients with displaced, off-ended, laterally angulated (>10°) or multiple fractures should be admitted for fracture reduction and fixation (K-wires or plates) under GA. This is particularly true for patients with deformity on the lateral projection.

### *Fifth metacarpal*

Virtually all fractures of the fifth metacarpal can be treated conservatively and followed up in a week if there is no rotational deformity and function is preserved. The neck is most commonly injured. The usual cause is throwing a punch.

Angulation of more than 45° or a significant reduction in the range of movement of the metacarpophalangeal joint may be an indication for surgery. This is best performed in theatre under GA, as a K-wire or plate may be used to hold the reduction. Discuss these cases with your registrar and admit if necessary.

Check the skin over the dorsae of the metacarpophalangeal joints carefully for evidence of laceration from an opponent's teeth ('fight bite'). All patients with such lacerations need to be admitted for exploration and washout of the joint under GA within 24 hours. Intravenous antibiotics are essential, and these should cover anaerobes as well as skin flora, for example benzylpenicillin, flucloxacillin and metronidazole.

Fractures of the shaft of the fifth metacarpal are again mainly treated conservatively with a backslab for pain control if necessary. If angulation is marked, however, apply traction and local pressure followed by a well-moulded backslab. This can be performed in the emergency department with analgesia and local infiltration. Displaced fractures can be reduced in the same way, but, if unsuccessful, admission for open reduction should be considered, as intervening soft tissue may be preventing the reduction.

Rarely, the base of the fifth metacarpal is dislocated. The patient should be admitted overnight for elevation of the hand and discussed with the registrar on admission. Obtain consent from the patient for closed reduction and possibly K-wire fixation under GA on the next trauma list.

**Key management points**

- Isolated, closed, undisplaced fractures: conservative treatment, mobilization, hand clinic in one week
- Closed, displaced, angulated or rotated fractures: admit for reduction and fixation under GA
- Open fractures: admit; intravenous antibiotics, irrigation, reduction and fixation under GA within 24 hours
- Fractures of neck of fifth metacarpal: conservative treatment
- 'Fight bites': admit for intravenous antibiotics and joint washout under GA

## Fractures and dislocations of the thumb

Fractures of the distal phalanx are managed in a similar way to fractures of the fingers. Dislocations of the interphalangeal joint should be reduced as soon as possible under a ring block with traction. Immobilize in a splint or POP, arrange a repeat radiograph and bring back to the hand clinic within the week. Fractures of the proximal phalanx are managed as for the fingers.

Dislocation of the metacarpophalangeal joint is relatively common and usually caused by a hyperextension injury. You should reduce these yourself as soon as possible. Administer a ring block; local infiltration is also helpful. Wait approximately 10–15 minutes and then reduce by applying traction, hyperextension and pressure over the metacarpophalangeal joint. Document the neurovascular status before and after reduction. As with the fingers, admit the patient overnight for elevation or discuss the patient with your registrar, ideally while the ring block is still in effect. Closed reduction can fail; if it does, admit for urgent open reduction. After successful reduction, put into a thumb spica, which immobilizes the metacarpophalangeal joint but allows proximal interphalangeal motion. Carpometacarpal dislocations occur more rarely, but they should be managed in the same way.

Metacarpal fractures in the thumb can be treated conservatively with splinting if angulation is acceptable. As for the fingers, assess the range of motion; if motion is impaired significantly, surgery may be indicated. Fractures of the thumb base include Bennett's and Rolando's fractures, both of which are intra-articular fractures that need reduction and internal fixation. Discuss all fractures of the thumb base with your registrar, because a significant minority will need fixation to achieve an acceptable position. It is worth discussing all thumb fractures (apart from those of the terminal phalanx) with your registrar because of their relative rarity and the importance of the thumb in the function of the hand.

## *Gamekeeper's thumb*

Gamekeeper's thumb is a rupture of the ulnar collateral ligament of the metacarpophalangeal joint of the thumb. It is caused by hyperabduction of the thumb and is diagnosed by tenderness over the ulna aspect of the joint and laxity when the ligament is stressed. It often is necessary to infiltrate the area with local anaesthetic to fully test the laxity. Discuss these patients with your registrar, as some patients are suitable for acute repair of the ulnar collateral ligament. Otherwise, patients with these injuries should be put into a cast or thumb spica and given an appointment at the next hand clinic.

**Key management points**

- Terminal phalanx fractures: treat as per fingers
- Proximal phalanx/metacarpal fractures:
  - Closed, undisplaced, stable fractures: conservative treatment, mobilize, hand clinic in one week
  - Closed unstable fractures: admit for reduction and fixation under GA
- Thumb base fractures: discuss with registrar, admit if intra-articular for reduction and K-wire/internal fixation under GA
- Open fractures: admit; intravenous antibiotics; irrigation, reduction and fixation under GA within 24 hours
- Dislocations: reduce immediately under ring block, admit for possible exploration and stabilization under GA

## *Fractures and dislocations of the carpal bones*

Fractures and dislocations of the carpal bones are uncommon injuries, but they are easily missed, which can have serious consequences. Suspect such injuries in patients who have experienced high-energy injuries and have gross swelling and tenderness of the carpus. Even if you cannot see a carpal fracture or dislocation in these cases, review the radiograph with your registrar, as these injuries can be difficult to spot. Scaphoid fractures have been specifically excluded from this chapter, as they are traditionally managed by orthopaedic surgeons; however, it is wise to keep them in mind.

Fractures of the carpal bones, unless displaced, can be treated conservatively in a cast and reviewed in the next hand clinic. Admit patients with displaced carpal fractures for elevation and reduction and fixation under GA. Because of their rarity and seriousness, discuss all carpal fractures, suspected or otherwise, with your registrar at the time you see the patient or the next day.

Dislocations of the carpus may involve any of the carpal bones and include fractures. The most commonly affected bone is the lunate. The dislocation may be *perilunate*, in which the bones distal to the lunate are dislocated, or *lunate*, in which the lunate alone is dislocated volarly to the radius and the rest of the carpus. This is seen on the lateral views. Check the median nerve. These dislocations will need urgent closed or open reduction under GA in theatre whatever the time of day.

**Key management points**

- Suspected carpal injury, no fracture: conservative treatment, early hand clinic appointment, get radiographs reviewed
- Undisplaced: conservative treatment, early appointment in hand clinic
- Displaced carpal fractures: admit for reduction and fixation under GA
- Dislocations: check neurovascular status, admit for urgent reduction under GA, call registrar
- Open fractures: admit; intravenous antibiotics; irrigation, reduction and fixation under GA within 24 hours

## Summary

Hand fractures are common and often can be treated conservatively unless the patient has a functional deficit, intra-articular involvement, multiple fractures or a severe soft-tissue injury. Early diagnosis and prompt treatment is the key to restoring function. Intervention is needed in fractures that involve angulation or rotation, intra-articular fractures, open fractures or inherently unstable fractures.

**Key management points**

- Check for neurovascular compromise
- Reduce dislocations
- Elevate
- Closed and stable fractures: splint or POP, next hand clinic with radiographs taken on arrival
- Closed and unstable fractures: admit for surgery next list (GA)
- Open fractures: admit for surgery next list (GA), intravenous antibiotics
- Portable radiograph machine for theatre
- Ensure follow-up in hand clinic with radiographs taken on arrival (give the patient a form)

# Crush injuries

Specific problems with crush injuries of the hand are the difficulty in determining the degree of viability and control of oedema. Oedema tends to worsen with time, and the extreme endpoint of this can be compartment syndrome. Crush injuries are also often associated with compound fractures. In crush injuries, there is no clear demarcation between normal and contused tissues. Although fractures are common, tendons and nerves usually escape division, but they may be contused.

It is often impossible to be precise about the vitality of crushed tissues. Subcutaneous connective tissues are devitalized more easily than the skin, and their mistaken preservation may lead to secondary necrosis of the overlying skin. Important factors to consider are:

- presence or absence of bleeding from the cut skin edge
- degree of laceration of the tissues and contamination with foreign material
- direction of arterial supply and venous drainage in relation to avulsed flaps of skin
- length of time since injury
- first-aid treatment received.

A defect in venous drainage can cause oedema and is a factor in tissue necrosis. It is often inseparable from arterial insufficiency. Commonly both venous and arterial circulations are impaired. Tourniquets are usually avoided in theatre for crush injuries. Healing will probably be slow, and some tissue necrosis may occur. This cannot be avoided altogether, so primary repair of deep structures should be limited to stabilization of fractures.

The basic cause of oedema in the hand is defective venous and lymphatic drainage. Although the main arterial supply passes through the volar surface of the hand, the circulatory return is by the dorsum, and this will be impaired by all factors that obstruct or interfere with the pumping system of the muscles. These factors may be independent of the injury and include:

- immobility and lack of use
- constrictive dressing improperly applied
- dependent position of the arm
- unphysiological position of the hand – e.g. flexion of the wrist.

Although oedema can be caused by any injury to the hand, or indeed the rest of the limb, it often is associated with:

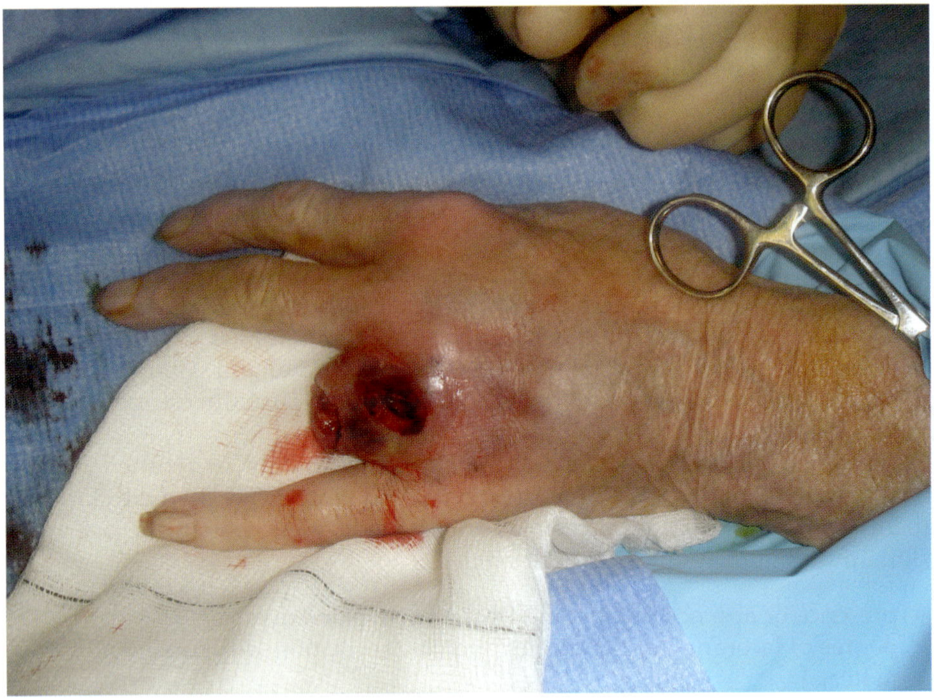

**Figure 1.24** Amputation of a digit after a crush injury

- deep laceration across the back of the wrist, which divides the venous channels
- crush injuries (contusion and thrombosis of larger vessels cause a circulatory disturbance that is further aggravated by extravasation of fluid because of capillary damage).

Increased swelling limits active movements of the digits, which leads to persistent oedema. This eventually causes fibrosis and subcutaneous thickening, shortening of the ligaments, contracture of the capsules of the joints and, finally, 'frozen' hand.

Measures to control oedema include:

- avoiding sutures under tension
- care in the application of dressings
- elevation of the limb
- frequent active exercises

**Key management points**

- Admit for exploration and decompression under GA
- Elevate
- Urgent registrar review
- Watch for compartment syndrome

# Replants and revascularizations

A revascularization procedure differs from a replantation (Figures 1.25 and 1.26) in that the digit or limb remains attached to the body but its vascular supply has been divided. When taking a telephone referral for a replant, you need to ask the following questions:

- Which digit(s) or limb(s) is(are) affected?
- Which is the dominant hand?
- At what level is the amputation?
- At exactly what time did the injury occur?
- What is the mechanism of injury – clean laceration or crush?
- Where is the amputated part? What state is it in (is it worth replanting)?
- What colour is the digit distal to the injury and what is the capillary refill time (for revascularizations)?
- What other injuries does the patient have?
- What is the patient's previous medical history?
- Does the patient smoke? If so, how much?
- What is the patient's occupation and do they have any relevant hobbies?
- When did they last eat or drink?

It is worth discussing each case with your registrar before accepting the patient, as you may be unaware of reasons why the patient cannot be taken into theatre with the urgency required or the registrar may want to discuss it with their consultant, who may have to come in to the hospital. You should also bear in mind any other patients who are awaiting urgent surgery or are already in surgery.

Each patient must be assessed on an individual basis, but, roughly speaking, the indications for replantation of a digit are:

- multiple finger amputations
- thumb amputations
- hand amputations at the palm or wrist
- paediatric amputations.

Less absolute indications for replantation are:

- loss of a single digit, excluding the thumb
- ring avulsion injuries.

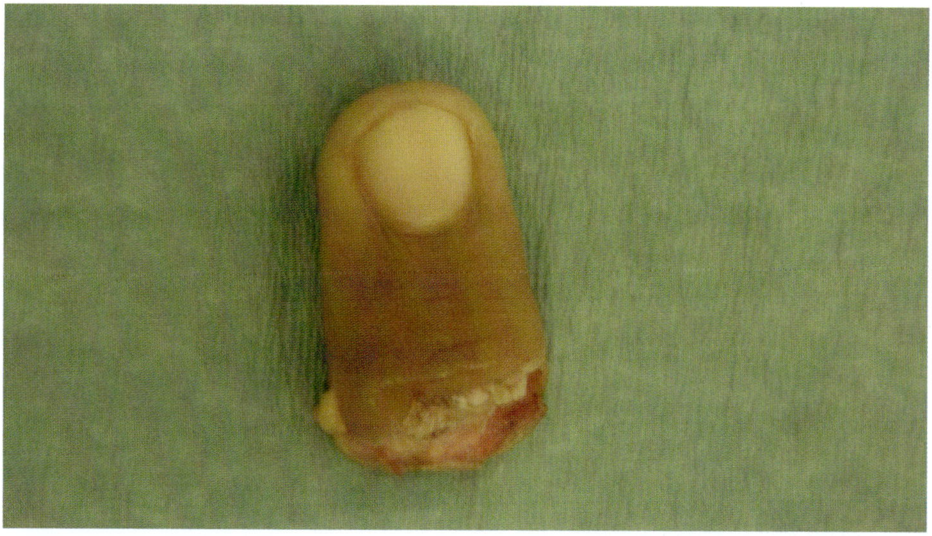

**Figure 1.25** Amputated digit

If you accept the patient, ask the referring doctor to put the amputated part in a saline-soaked sterile swab inside a sterile bag that itself is placed in a bag of ice. Essentially, the part should be kept cold but not in direct contact with ice, which will damage it. The patient should be kept nil by mouth, and both patient and part should be transferred to your hospital under blue lights. A digit is worth replanting within six hours of injury; after this, success is unlikely. Prepare theatre in the meantime. Be aware that a replant takes four hours or more.

Postoperatively, manage the patient as if they have had a small free flap, which effectively is what they have had. The patient and digit must be kept warm and well perfused with intravenous fluids and a urine output of at least 0.5 ml/kg/hr. Look out for arterial compromise (cold or white pallor) or venous congestion (blue pallor, rapid capillary refill). These are managed by re-exploration and leeches, respectively. In both cases, you should call your registrar immediately.

## Consent for replantation or revascularization

The complications are as for other operations for hand trauma, as well as the following:

- Prolonged GA
- Repair of nerves, vessels, muscles and/or tendons

- Vein grafts (small veins harvested from hand or forearm)
- Replantation failure (vessels may be too damaged or simply will not flow)
- Terminalization
- Internal fixation, K-wires
- Necrosis (total or partial)
- Venous congestion and leeches
- Cold intolerance
- Numbness
- Poor function
- Amputation of replanted digit if it turns out be non-functional or painful.

**Key management points**

- Transfer under blue lights
- Surgery as soon as possible but within six hours
- Correct transport of amputated part
- Intravenous infusion of antibiotics
- Manage postoperatively as if it was a free flap (see page 115)

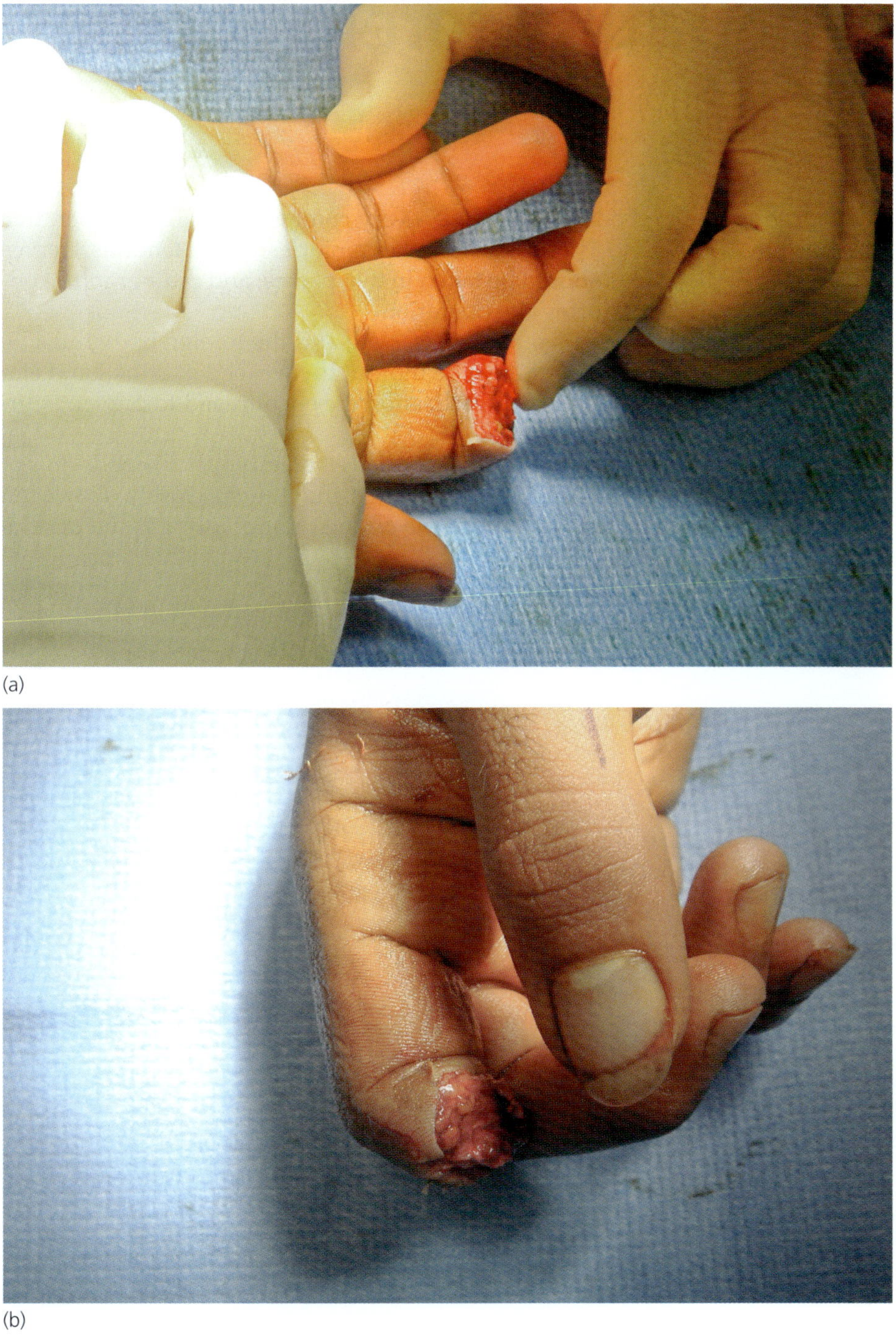

(a)

(b)

**Figure 1.26** Proximal stump of amputated digit: (a) volar and (b) lateral view

# Penetrating foreign bodies

A penetrating foreign body in the hand is very common. Careful preoperative examination of the hand is essential to assess injuries to the tendons, nerves and vessels. Radiographs should be taken in two planes, and radiographic control should be available during the operation.

The patient's tetanus status must be assessed, and the foreign body must be removed in theatre. The wound must be thoroughly washed and the hand elevated. Antibiotic cover and early mobilization are encouraged to prevent stiffness.

Be aware that some foreign bodies, especially some types of wood, do not show on radiographs, so you should examine the patient closely. However, even if the foreign body itself is not visible on the radiograph, a tissue disruption or air may be visible.

# Extravasation injuries

An extravasation injury results from leakage of solutions from veins to surrounding tissue spaces during intravenous administration. These injuries result in significant morbidity that vary with the particular agent, including severe disfigurement, functional loss and amputation. Initial symptoms include pain and burning at the catheter site. Oedema is followed by skin blistering and eventual sloughing at 5–7 days. The hand or extremity may seem cool and cyanotic during this time. Painful, full-thickness skin ulcerations occur, which can become infected and can culminate in sepsis (Figure 1.27). Other less common features are compartment syndrome, nerve compression, permanent nerve deficits, sympathetic dystrophy and permanent joint stiffness.

Commonly used chemotherapeutic agents are toxic locally after extravasation. Other agents known to produce severe tissue necrosis are phenytoin, noradrenaline, dopamine, albumin, lipid agents and solutions that contain hypertonic dextrose or calcium salts. Consult the *British National Formulary* for individual agents.

Factors that determine the degree of tissue damage from an extravasation injury are:

- type of agent (i.e. vesicant versus irritant or non-vesicant)
- site of extravasation
- concentration and dose of vesicant
- host response
- delay in recognition and initiation of treatment
- type of treatment.

Treatment consists of stopping the infusion and removing the catheter, followed by application of a light dressing. The extremity is splinted for comfort and protection and elevated. An ice pack is applied to the site of extravasation and surrounding tissues.

If the agent is vesicant, multiple punctures over the affected area and irrigation to dilute the content with normal saline are recommended. Following demarcation, wide excision of all involved tissues to viable margins is recommended. Early rehabilitation, consisting of active range of motion exercises and oedema control, should be initiated to prevent residual stiffness.

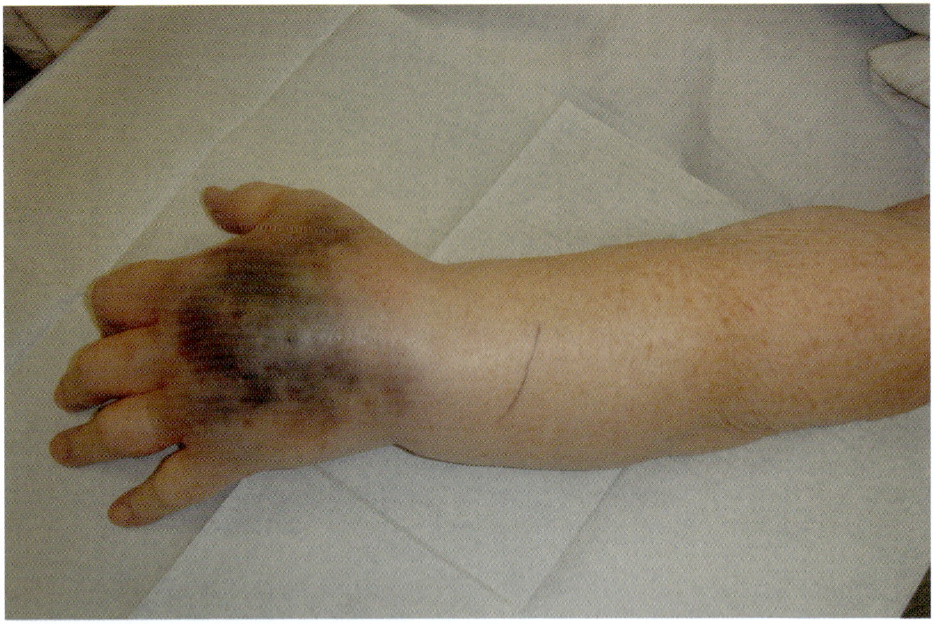

(a)

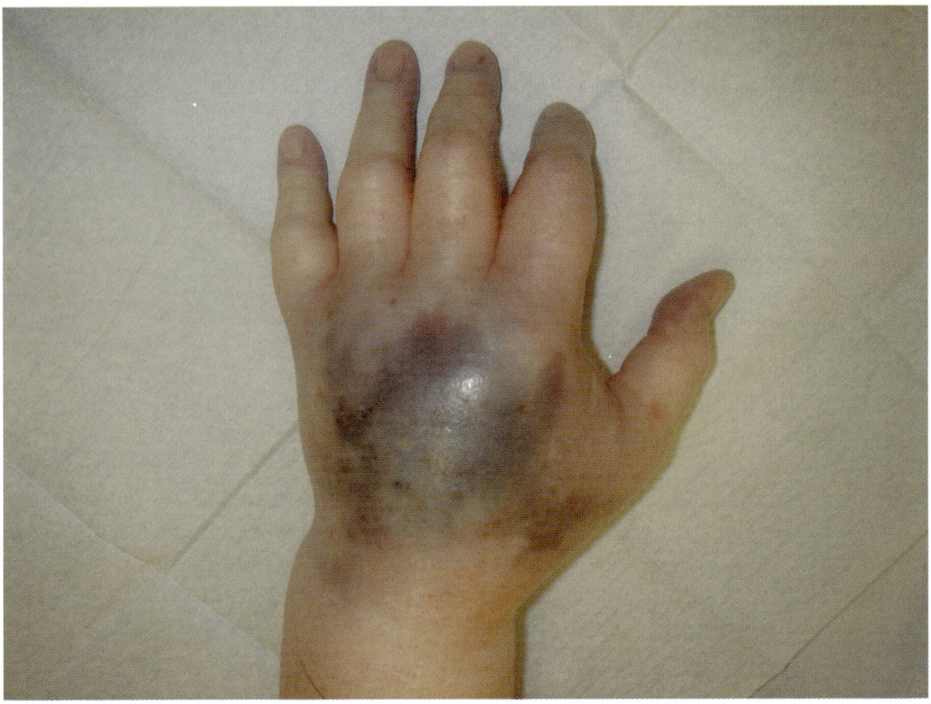

(b)

**Figure 1.27** Severe extravasation injury

**Key management points**

- Identify the involved agent
- Admit for irrigation under LA on ward or GA
- Elevate
- Observe for skin necrosis in next 48 hours

# High-pressure injection injuries

A high-pressure injection injury is the accidental innoculation of a foreign material or substance into the hand or digit via a pressurized industrial device such as a paint or spray gun. The most common site is the tip of the non-dominant index finger.

The patient may complain only of a stinging or burning sensation, and the appearance of the hand or finger may seem relatively innocuous. Within hours, the area becomes swollen, pale, numb and painful. A small entrance wound may be noted. If unrecognized or inappropriately treated, ischaemia and tissue necrosis ensue and can culminate in bacterial infection and gangrene. The patient may become febrile as a result of systemic absorption of the injected material, with leukocytosis, lymphangitis or lymphadenitis.

Critical information to obtain includes:

- time of injury
- type of material injected
- location of entrance wound
- presence of infection, ischaemia or gangrene.

This is a surgical emergency that requires recognition and appropriate treatment. Radiographs can locate any radio-opaque material that can guide the extent of the surgical approach. Broad-spectrum antibiotics should be initiated.

Surgical technique includes wide exposure, debridement of all devitalized tissues and injected material, preservation of neurovascular structures, pulsed lavage irrigation, drainage and open packing. Serial debridements are performed at intervals of 48–72 hours, as necessary, and are followed by delayed primary wound closure or healing by secondary intention. Early motion is important, and amputation may be necessary in patients who present late.

Factors associated with poor prognosis and increased risk of subsequent amputation include:

- delay in treatment
- injection of oil-based solvent such as grease, paint or paint thinner
- injection into the finger
- high injection pressure
- high volume of injected material.

**Key management points**

- Identify the involved agent
- Admit for urgent exploration and debridement under GA
- Elevate
- Intravenous broad-spectrum antibiotics

# Deliberate self-harm

The surgical management of injuries sustained from deliberate self-harm (DSH) does not differ from that for injuries sustained ordinarily, except in the case of multiple repeats of self-harm (Figure 1.28), for example, which may make further tendon repairs pointless. In general, however, it is better to see the patient and then make this decision rather than to reject the referral outright.

The main reason for mentioning injuries caused by DSH is that you must insist the referring hospital arranges for the patient to be seen by a psychiatrist before transfer, and you must hear the outcome of that assessment before you accept the patient. The psychiatrist usually finds that the patient is safe enough to be transferred without an accompanying psychiatric trained nurse and arranges a follow-up appointment after discharge from plastic surgery. Occasionally, however, the patient is still deemed to represent a considerable risk to themselves in terms of further self-harm or suicide. In such cases, accept the patient only if the referring hospital is going to provide psychiatric nursing

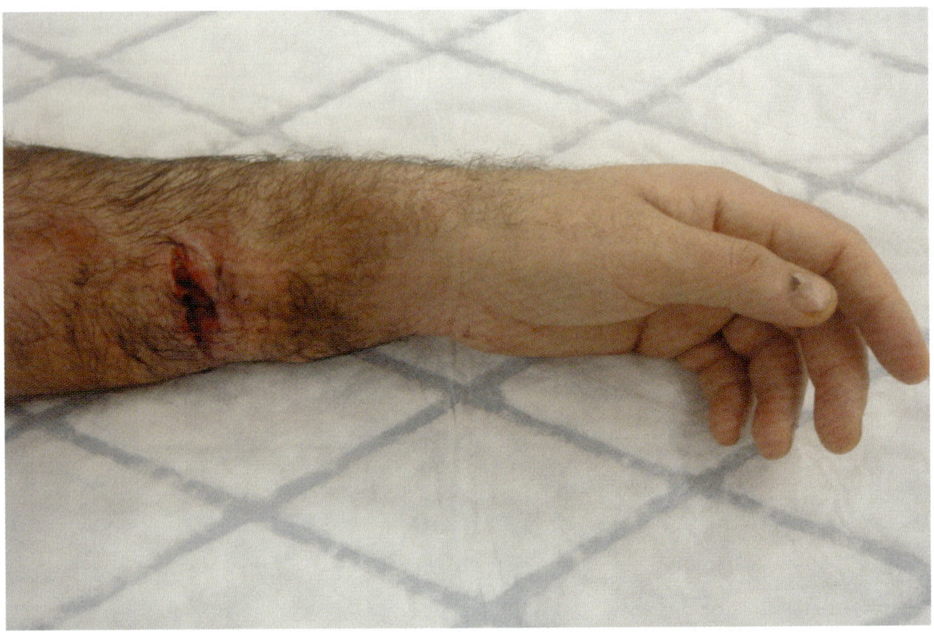

**Figure 1.28** Laceration after deliberate self-harm

cover for the patient around the clock until discharge. If a patient is acutely psychiatrically unwell in any other way, it is advisable to insist on a similar level of nursing cover for them as well.

The aim of this approach is to make sure that you and your ward staff are responsible only for the patient's welfare in terms of plastic surgery and that the psychiatric team take full responsibility for the patient's psychological welfare.

**Key management points**

- Treat injuries caused by DSH as you would any other injury
- Psychiatric assessment with known outcome and follow-up arranged before transfer
- Patient to be accompanied by 24-hour psychiatric nurse if appropriate
- Consider missed overdoses

# Consent for patients with hand trauma

Several complications or likely occurrences are common to all operations to repair hand trauma such as infections, complications related to general anaesthetic, scars and stiffness (Table 1.8). In addition, there are complications that are specific to the operation such as tendon rerupture, neuromas, graft failure and donor site scars. Splints and hand therapy are not strictly speaking complications, but putting them down on the form reminds you to warn patients of these likely occurrences.

**Table 1.8** Complications associated with operations for hand injuries.

| Type of operation | Complication |
|---|---|
| All | • Scarring<br>• Infection<br>• Bleeding<br>• Possible repair of nerves, vessels, muscles and/or tendons<br>• Stiffness<br>• Splints<br>• General anaesthesia |
| Tendon operations | • Tendon rerupture |
| Nerve repairs | • Neuromas<br>• No or incomplete recovery of sensation or movement |
| Nail-bed injuries | • Abnormal or absent nail growth |
| Local flaps and composite grafts | • Necrosis |
| Split and full-thickness grafts | • Graft failure<br>• Delayed healing of donor site<br>• Scarring |
| Fractures | • K-wires<br>• Internal or external fixation<br>• Delayed union<br>• Non-union |

**Key management points**

For any consent:

- describe the nature and severity of the injury to patient
- explain the treatment options
- propose the recommended treatment
- explain the risk factors (general and specific)
- explain the outcome and follow-up after treatment

# 2 Infections

The infections you will most commonly see in relation to plastic surgery will be post-traumatic and post-surgical wound infections and cellulitis. The infections you must be on guard for are joint infections and open fractures (particularly after 'fight-bites'), burn infections (these can rapidly progress to septic shock or toxic shock syndrome) and necrotizing fasciitis.

The principles of management for each are essentially the same: admission, wound swab and blood cultures, FBC/U&E/CRP, elevation, X-ray if indicated, early surgery if indicated. These patients must be reviewed regularly, your seniors should be informed and you must remember to specifically hand over these patients at the close of your shift.

# Hand infections

Infections of the hand are common and account for 20% of all admissions for hand injuries. Traumatic causes account for 60%, human bites for 30% and animal bites for 10%.

The aim of prompt treatment of hand infections is to restore optimal function in a short time. Delay in treatment can cause pain, stiffness and poor function, with possible amputation in extreme cases.

The most common pathogen in hand infections is *Staphylococcus aureus*, which causes a purulent infection 3–5 days after the event. A detailed history and examination is essential, however, as inadequate use of broad-spectrum antibiotics can cause unnecessary side-effects and complications to the patient, as well as the development of resistant strains.

Infections with a foul odour and purulent discharge usually require intravenous antibiotics as initial therapy. Meticulous wound debridement and care is preferred over the routine use of antibiotics in hand injuries.

Cellulitis is a common superficial infection that presents as erythema, swelling, pain and occasional lymphangitis. Treatment includes rest, elevation, splinting and antibiotics.

Management of hand infections can be summarized as:

- adequate drainage of all loculations of pus and debridement of necrotic tissue
- start with broad-spectrum antibiotics until sensitivities are known and then be guided by your microbiological colleagues and local guidelines
- prophylactic tetanus for all penetrating wounds
- rest, elevation and immobilization in a position of function
- early aggressive hand therapy.

## Immediate management

Immediate management involves the following:

- History
- Examination
- Assess whether or not immediate incision and washout is required – are there visible areas of pus?
- Elevate
- Antibiotics: oral or intravenous (find out the preference in your local hospital; co-amoxiclav or flucloxacillin)

- Review: infections get better or worse, so it is imperative that you observe, as they can spread rapidly (especially in cases involving streptococcal species) and can lead to necrotizing fasciitis.

**Key management points**

- Admit
- Swab if 'swabbable'
- Elevate
- Intravenous antibiotics, with or without tetanus
- Abscess: book for incision and drainage under GA
- Ensure follow-up in dressing clinic 24–48 hours after discharge

# Paronychia

Paronychia is an infection of the structures that surround the proximal and lateral nail. It begins as erythema, swelling and discomfort at the nail fold, sometimes with fluctuation and frank pus (Figure 2.1).

If detected early, warm soaks, elevation and oral antibiotics may be sufficient; however, if the infection has been present for more than 24 hours or fluctuation is detected under the nail, the nail fold must be elevated and pus drained. More aggressive drainage is warranted if the infection extends proximally to the nail fold. If treated inadequately, the pus may extend to the ventral surface (Figure 2.1), in which case the pressure from the accumulated pus can permanently damage the germinal matrix.

**Key management points**

- Elevate
- Admit for incision and drainage and removal of nail under LA
- Intravenous antibiotics
- Discharge to home with oral antibiotics
- Review in 24 hours

## Infections of the pulp space (felons)

Longitudinal septa in the pulp anchor the tip of the distal phalanx. In the presence of infection, these septa can compartmentalize and prevent drainage. Infections of the pulp space (felons; Figure 2.3) usually occur as a result of penetrating trauma. Radiographic investigations are required to assess for any foreign bodies. The most common pathogen is *Staphylococcus aureus,* but Gram-negative organisms also have been reported.

It is important to take a thorough history from patients, looking particularly for diabetes or immunosuppression. The patient usually presents with red swollen pulp and complains of a severe throbbing pain, especially when the finger is dependent, because of increased tissue pressure that essentially causes compartment syndrome of the pulp.

If the felon is detected early, incision and drainage followed by elevation and oral antibiotics usually is sufficient. In advanced states, the blood supply to the pulp can be compromised, which results in soft tissue necrosis, tenosynovitis, septic arthritis and even osteomyelitis. The usual site of drainage is where the

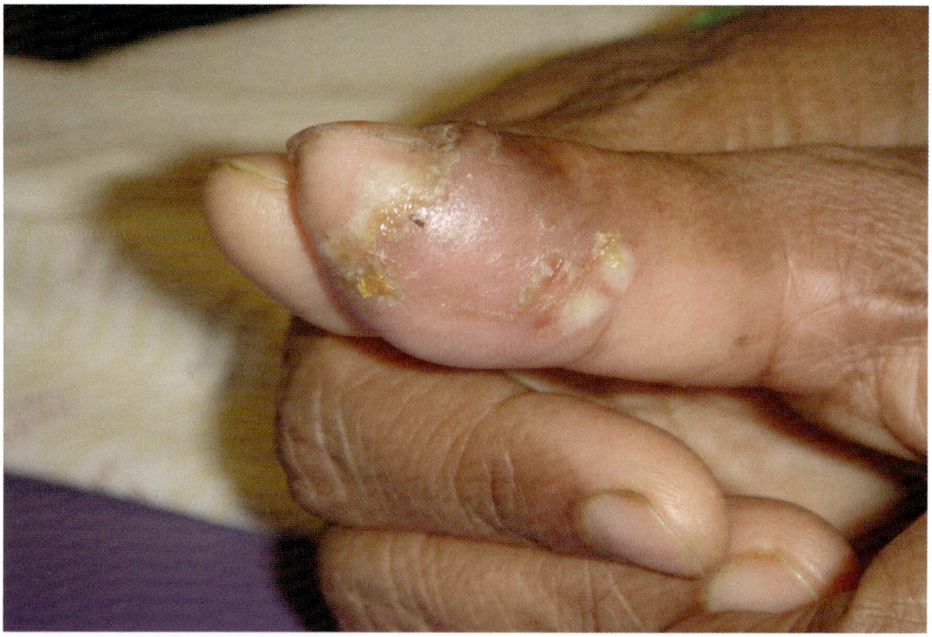

(a)

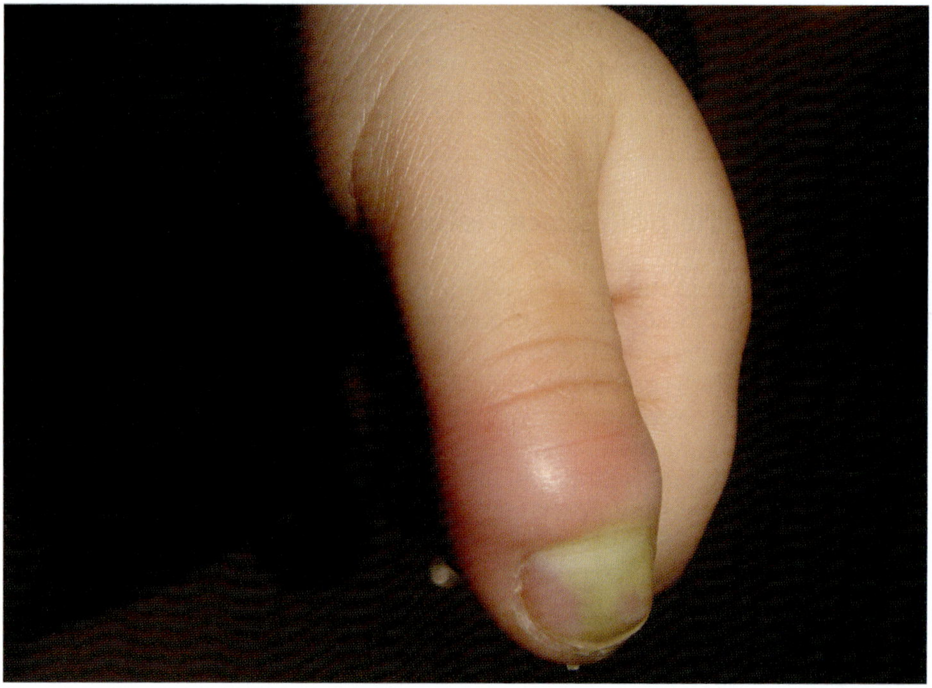

(b)

**Figure 2.1** Paronychia: (a) lateral and (b) dorsal view

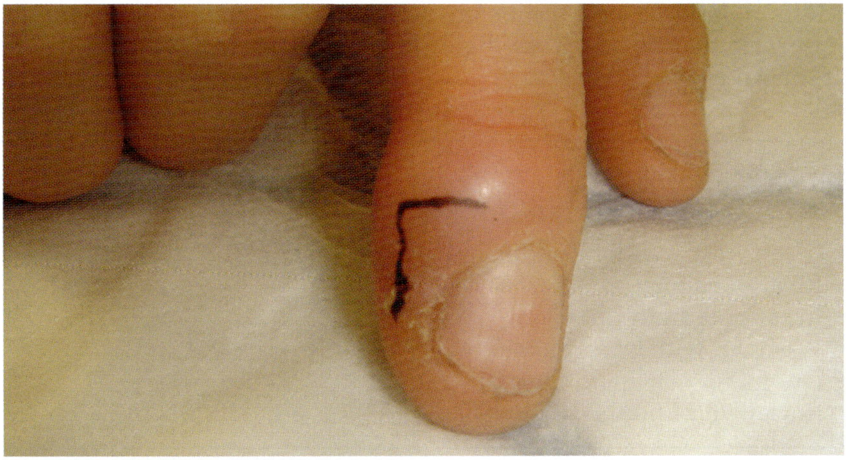

**Figure 2.2** Paronychia with incision marked

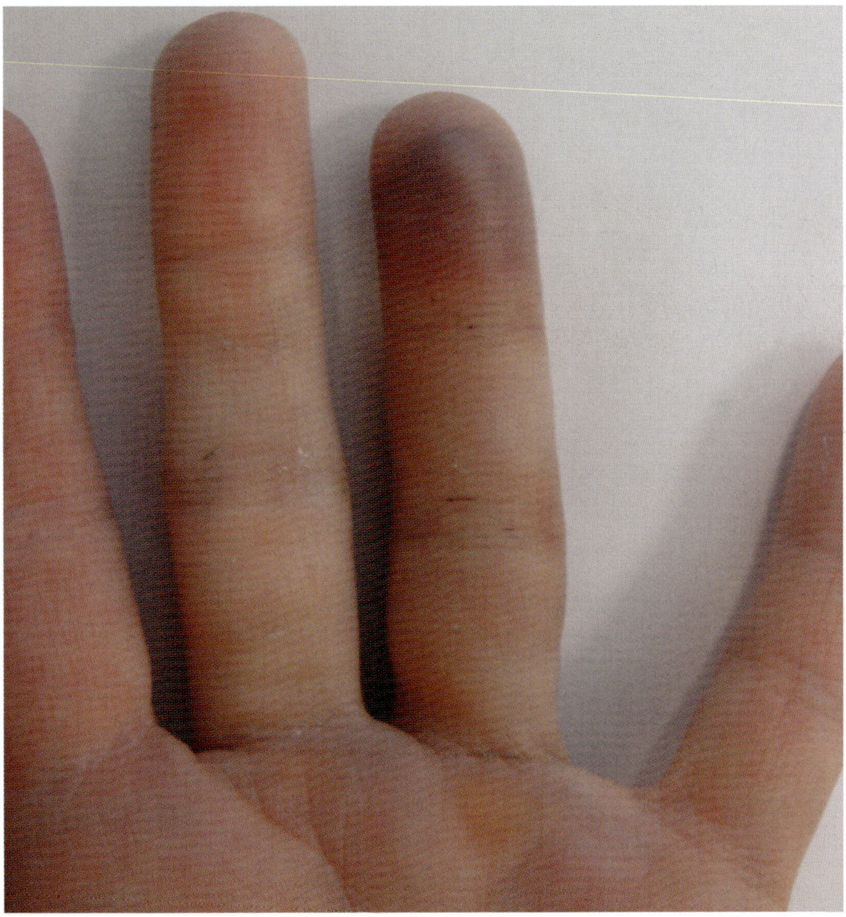

**Figure 2.3** A felon

abscess is pointing. Good results are seen with longitudinal incisions on the volar surface that do not cross the distal interphalangeal joint. This incision tends to heal well.

**Key management points**

- Ring block
- Clean with povidone iodine or chlorhexidine
- Ring tourniquet
- Incise and drain
- Wash out with *lots* of saline
- Dress
- Review in 24 hours

# Flexor tendon sheath infections

Flexor tendon sheath infection is an infection of the sheath that forms the gliding surface around the flexor tendons in the hand. Infection can destroy the delicate gliding surfaces of the tendon sheaths, resulting in a stiff and painful finger. This is an emergency and a delay in or inappropriate treatment can lead to devastating consequences. Prolonged delay in treatment can cause rupture of the sheath, with spread of infection to palm spaces, as well as ischaemic rupture of the tendon itself.

Most cases of flexor tendon sheath infection are caused by a penetrating trauma. The main causative organism is *Staphylococcus aureus*. Four cardinal signs have been described for flexor tendon sheath infection (Figure 2.4):

- fusiform swelling of the digit
- partially flexed posture of the digit
- tenderness along the entire flexor tendon sheath
- pain along the entire flexor sheath with passive extension.

When the diagnosis is uncertain, ultrasound can be used to show swelling of the tendon, as well as pretendinous fluid. Diagnosis can be confirmed at the time of surgery by aspiration of the flexor sheath. Once the diagnosis is made, treatment of surgical drainage must be initiated promptly. An active range of motion exercises is begun with the first dressing change on the ward.

**Immediate management (EMERGENCY)**

- History and examination
- Admit
- Consent for theatre under GA
- Swab if 'swabbable', intravenous cultures if pyrexial
- Full blood count and C-reactive protein
- Intravenous broad-spectrum antibiotics
- Elevate in a Bradford sling
- Book the next available emergency theatre session – DO NOT wait until the next day

**Key management points**

- Admit for emergency surgery
- Elevate
- Intravenous antibiotics

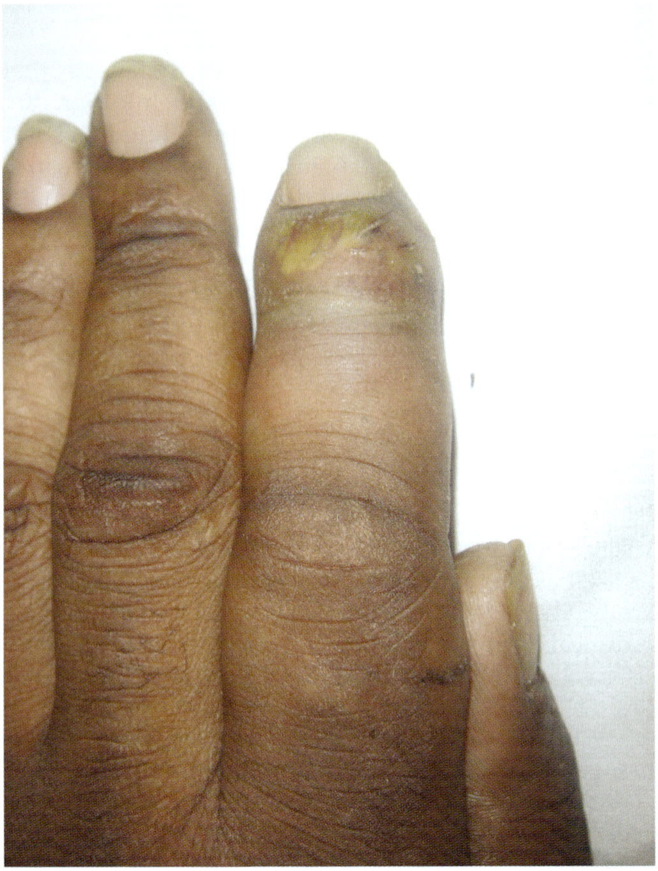

(a)

**Figure 2.4** Signs of flexor tendon sheath infection on two different fingers: (a) dorsal view (*continued*)

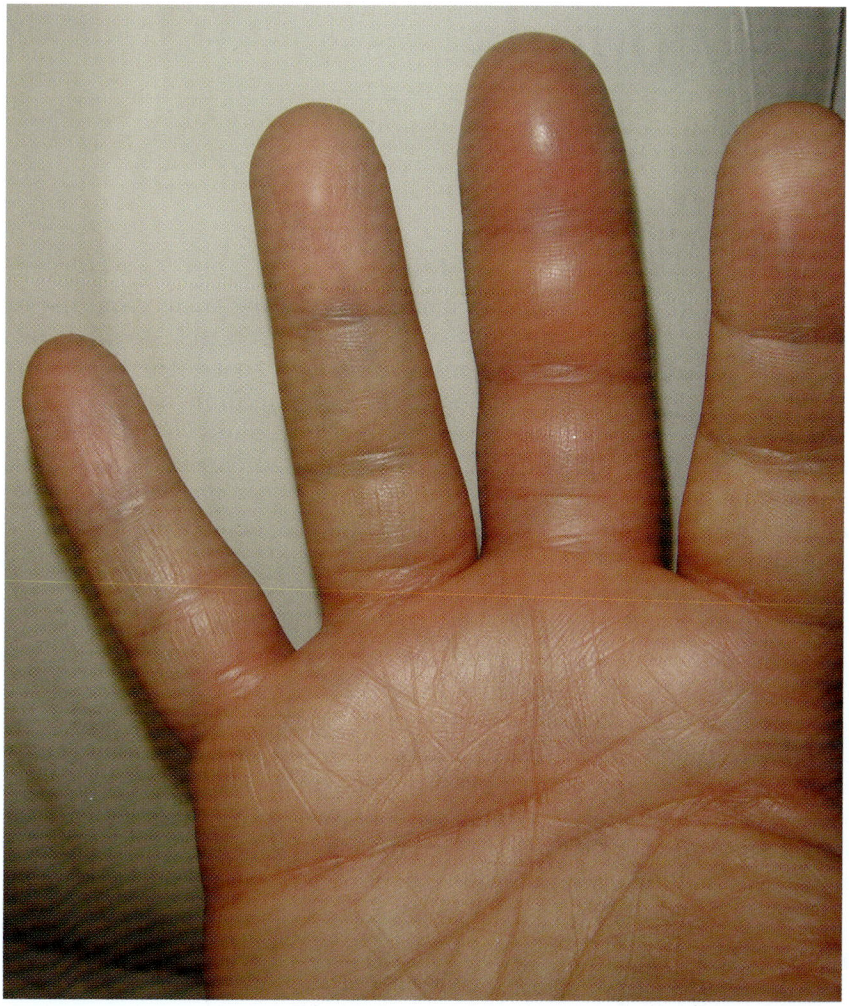

(b)

**Figure 2.4** (*continued*) Signs of flexor tendon sheath infection on two different fingers: (b) volar view

# Bite wounds

## Human ('fight') bites

Most bites to the hand are human bites. For example, a clenched fist injury occurs when the fist strikes the mouth of another person and a tooth penetrates the skin and often the underlying metacarpal joint space. The hand must be assessed in the clenched fist position to allow an accurate assessment of the depth of injury. Radiological investigation may show a fracture of the metacarpal head, air in the joints and occasionally a foreign body, such as a broken tooth (delayed presentation may show early signs of early osteomyelitis). After a few days, the infection can manifest as a red, swollen, painful hand with occasional lymphangitis and regional lymphadenitis. The patient may have systemic symptoms.

Most cultures yield *Staphylococcus aureus* and *Streptococcus viridans*. Other organisms commonly encountered are anaerobic *Bacteroides* species and *Eikenella corrodens*, which is sensitive to penicillin.

The clenched fist wound to the metacarpophalangeal joint is a notoriously underestimated and undertreated injury. All cases should be managed with splinting, elevation, antibiotics and surgical exploration. If infection is established, irrigation of the joint may be continued postoperatively for up to 72 hours. Early motion (after 48–72 hours) should be advocated, as stiffness is one of the more difficult complications to treat.

## Animal bites

### *Dog bites*

Domestic dog bites account for 90% of all animal bites. Dog bites become infected less often than human or cat bites, but a dog's powerful jaw can devitalize tissues. The resulting wound can be a puncture, laceration, avulsion or crush, or their combination (Figure 2.5). As with human bites, the most common pathogens are usually a mixture of aerobes (for example, *Staphylococcus aureus* and *Streptococcus viridans*), anaerobes (various *Bacteroides* species) and *Pasteurella multocida*.

The area should be irrigated thoroughly with normal saline, the wound margins sharply excised and the wound edges loosely approximated with sutures. The tetanus status of the patient and the rabies status of the animal should be verified, and further vaccinations administered as appropriate. Secondary closure may be required in severe cases.

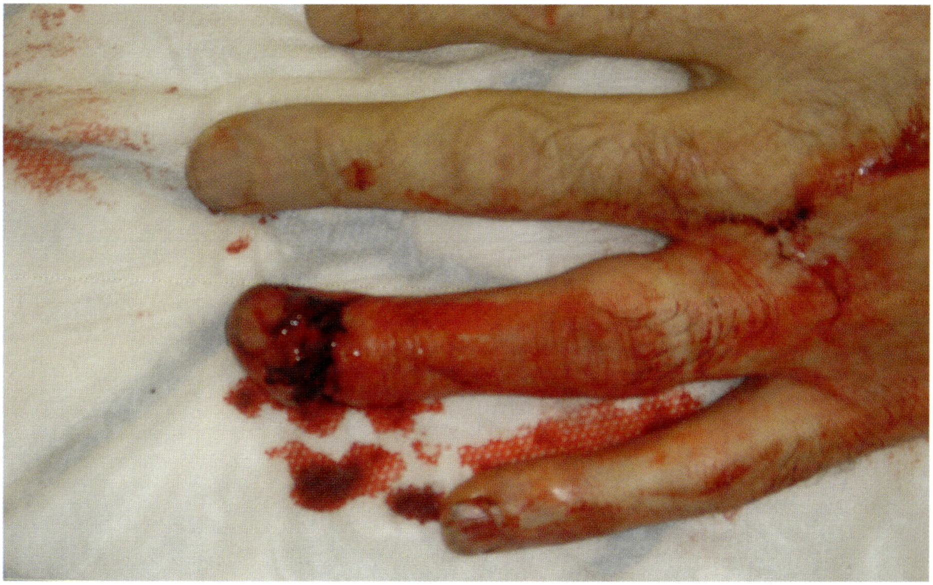

**Figure 2.5** Patient who has been bitten by a dog

## *Cat bites*

Domestic cat bites account for 5% of animal-bite wounds to the hand. Cat's teeth are long and sharp, and the injury they inflict tends to be a deep puncture wound. The wound should be irrigated and loosely approximated if large enough to warrant suturing, and antibiotic cover should be given.

Cat bites may also give rise to cat-scratch fever, an infection caused by an intracellular Gram-negative rod. The primary lesion is a small pustule or furuncle with surrounding oedema at the site of a cat scratch or bite. A similar lesion is seen at the regional lymph nodes. The course of the disease is benign and self-limiting, and treatment is symptomatic. The incubation period is 1–2 weeks and the symptoms last up to three weeks, although the adenopathy typically lasts six weeks and occasionally years.

**Immediate management**

- History and examination
- Radiography to check for fractures
- Local anaesthesia or regional block if appropriate
- Wash with normal saline or povidone iodine
- Elevate
- Dress appropriately
- Antibiotics
- Review

**Key management points**

- Bite wounds need surgical exploration
- Admit for GA
- Intravenous antibiotics
- Elevation
- Early follow-up

# Necrotizing fasciitis

Necrotizing fasciitis is a synergistic necrotizing bacterial infection of the subcutaneous tissues that, if untreated, may cause extensive tissue necrosis or death within hours. A number of bacteria can cause this condition, but the most common culprits are group A haemolytic streptococci. Necrotizing fasciitis presents as skin discoloration anywhere on the body, may spread rapidly within hours and can be accompanied by systemic signs of infection. The initial rash may be very small and innocuous, but if this is accompanied by fever, pain and worsening malaise, you must consider this diagnosis. Patients who are at particular risk of developing this infection are those with diabetes, immunocompromised patients, 'down and outs' (e.g. people with alcoholism, homeless people, people with drug addictions, etc.) , patients with wounds from 'contaminated' surgery (e.g. bowel surgery, gynaecological surgery, surgery for trauma) and patients who are generally unwell. Fit and healthy individuals may be affected, however, and a history of trauma preceding the onset is not essential.

If you ever even minutely suspect necrotizing fasciitis, you must immediately ask your registrar to see the patient urgently and in the meantime prepare the patient for imminent theatre. Mark the margins of the rash. Administer oxygen to the patient and insert two large calibre Venflon cannulae. Take blood for full blood count, urea and electrolytes, liver function tests, coagulation panel, glucose, C-reactive protein, blood cultures, and group and save. Start intravenous resuscitation.

Inform the anaesthetist, intensive treatment unit and theatre. Inform the relevant consultant as soon as the diagnosis is made. Obtain consent from the patient for extensive debridement beyond the margins of the rash and split-skin grafting, and warn the patient that they may be taken to the intensive treatment unit and that the diagnosis is very serious. Discuss the case with the microbiologist before theatre and be guided by them and your senior colleagues with respect to antibiotics.

Be wary of accepting the transfer of patients with preoperative necrotizing fasciitis from other hospitals, because immediate surgery is the treatment for necrotizing fasciitis and transfer will add significant delay. Discuss all possible referrals for necrotizing fasciitis with your registrar promptly. They may want to speak to the referring hospital directly or even go there in order to be present during the surgery. Initial debridement ideally should be performed at the first hospital, and the patient can be transferred (for reconstruction) once the fasciitis is arrested and the patient is stable. Transfer obviously is essential if the referring unit does not have a qualified surgeon available.

**Summary**

- Admit
- Inform registrar immediately
- Resuscitate
- Full set of bloods
- Arrange surgery as soon as possible

# 3

# Burns, facial and lower limb trauma

The degree to which burns, facial trauma and lower limb trauma contribute to your on-call work will depend on the unit in which you work. These injuries are looked after by specialized units, so they often are not taught at a junior level and hence are mismanaged at other units before transfer. Units that do manage these types of injuries often have their own protocols – familiarize yourself with them and keep a copy to hand. The following chapters aim to give you a guide to the safe management of patients affected by these types of injuries.

# Burns injuries

## Referral process

Before accepting a patient, check with the nurse in charge of the unit to make sure you have a suitable bed, including a bed in the intensive treatment unit if required. In the case of major burns, a registrar or consultant should be informed as soon as the referral is taken.

Occasionally, the burns centre is unable to take a patient because there are no available beds. You should discuss patients who are refused referral with the on-call consultant burns surgeon to see if other arrangements can be made.

If your unit has a protocol for faxing to referring units, do so and make sure appropriate treatment is initiated at the referring hospital to prevent delay. You may need to give advice on how the patient should be resuscitated (including formula) and to ask the unit to perform investigations and insert cannulae and catheters.

It is important to ensure safe transfer, as the patient is *your* responsibility once they leave the referring hospital.

## Admission process and assessment

When patients arrive, follow Figure 3.1 and assess the burns.

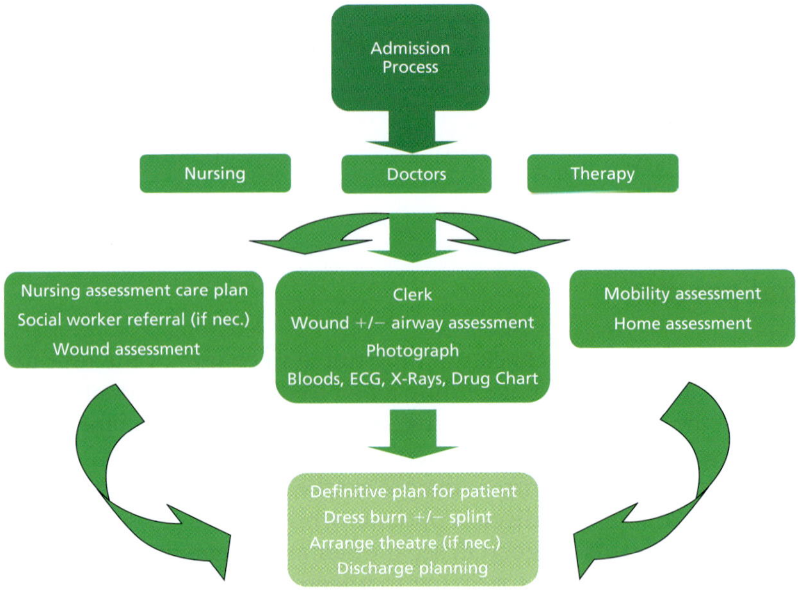


(a)

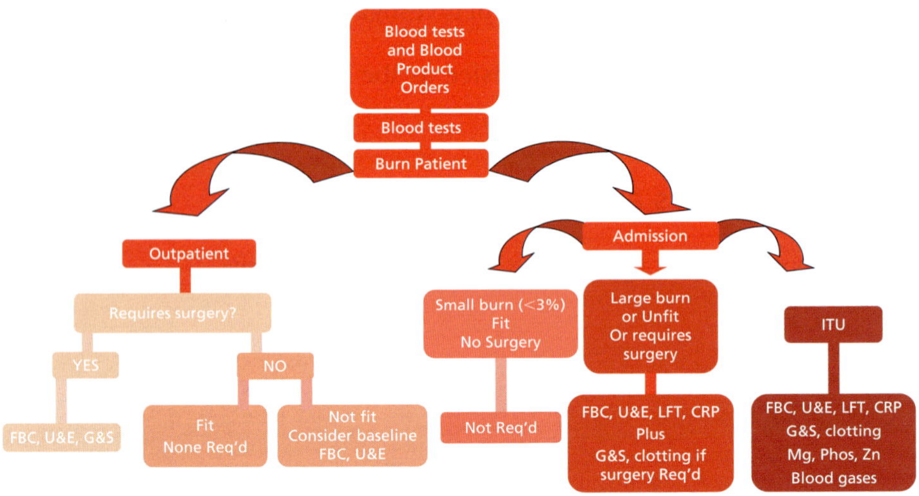


- ITU patients and larger burns to have bloods every day
- Ensure bloods are sent as early in the morning as possible
- Results to be documented the same day as taken and action taken as appropriate – SHO is responsible for this
- Consider amylase and tox screen for large burns
- Also baseline selenium and micronutrients should be performed in the early treatment period

(b)

**Figure 3.1** Admission process (a) and guide to investigations to be performed (b)

### *Depth and size of burn*

The two most important aspects to consider during burns assessment are the depth and size of the burn, which aid with management (Table 3.1). Other injuries, such as airway compromise, will be discussed later in this chapter. Photographs to document the extent of the burn injury must be taken for all new patients. Figure 3.2 shows the Lund and Browder chart, which is used to approximate the percentage burn; age-specific charts are used for children to reflect their different body proportions.

Laser Doppler machines measure the blood flow in burned areas and give a good guide as to whether or not a burn wound is likely to heal in two weeks. Laser Dopper is a very useful tool combined with clinical judgement and should be used in all cases when there is doubt about the true depth of a burn.

### *History*

Most burns will be referred from other hospitals. It is important to take a concise history as shown in Figure 3.3.

### *Airway*

In patients with major burns, look out for signs of airway compromise. These include:

- singing of nasal hairs
- oral soot
- carbonaceous sputum
- change of voice
- enclosed space.

**Table 3.1** Management of burns according to their depth and appearance.

| Depth | Appearance | Management |
|---|---|---|
| Superficial/ erythema | • Skin dry, intact and painful<br>• Blanches under pressure<br>• Minimal tissue damage<br>• Usually no blisters | • Requires no specific treatment |
| Superficial partial thickness | • Blisters immediately<br>• Wound bed normally pink/red<br>• Moist with moderate exudate<br>• Brisk capillary refill<br>• Very painful<br>• Sensitive to pain, air and temperature | • Conservative treatment with simple dressings – eg Jelonet, Mepitel or Telfa Clear, which require absorbent layer of gauze over them and a bandage or Mefix dressing to secure<br>• Smaller areas that are oozing less tissue fluid or those that are two or three days old may be treated with hydrocolloid or combination dressings such as Duoderm or Mepilex |
| Partial thickness/ deep dermal | • Red/pale white/creamy wound bed<br>• If blisters present, easy to separate, loose epidermis<br>• Sluggish capillary refill<br>• Slight pain but mostly insensate<br>• Sensitive to deep pressure but not pinprick | **Partial thickness**<br>• Likely to heal within 2–3 weeks<br>• Judgement is difficult<br>• If in doubt, senior review recommended<br>• Conservative therapy should be considered initially and Flammacerium usually is applied to create a firm, protective scar that is resistant to infection and preserves any remaining dermis<br>• If such burn wounds have failed to heal by two weeks, surgery should be considered<br>**Deep dermal**<br>• Usually require surgery at an early stage to preserve any remaining dermis<br>• Interim dressings usually consist of Flammacerium and Jelonet<br>• In a small number of cases, surgery is inappropriate for social or medical reasons, so Flammacerium should be continued<br>• Unless very small, all full thickness burns should be treated surgically<br>Interim dressings usually consist of Flammacerium and Jelonet |
| Full thickness | • White cream/cherry red wound bed<br>• Black/brown leathery eschar<br>• Minimal pain, if any<br>• Thrombosed vessels may be visible<br>• Insensate | |

BURN SHEET

Name ........................................................ AGE .................. NUMBER ...........................

BURN RECORD: AGES? TO ADULT. DATE OF OBSERVATION .....................................

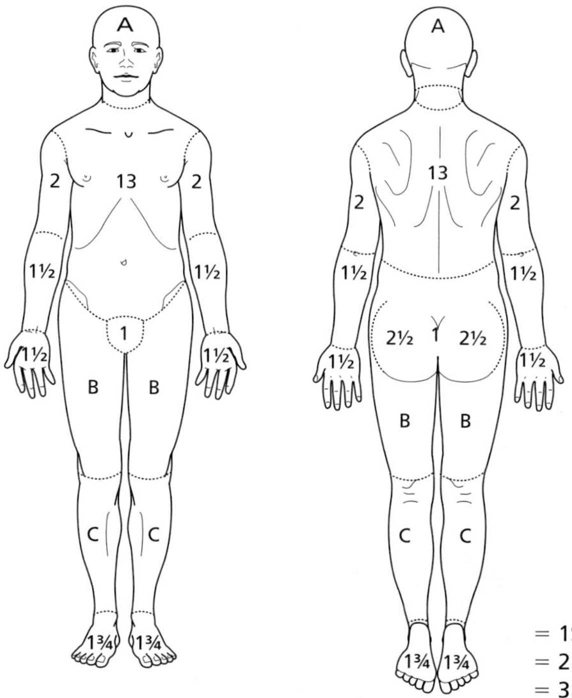


= 1ST DEGREE
= 2ND DEGREE
= 3RD DEGREE

RELATIVE PERCENTAGES OF AREAS AFFECTED BY GROWTH

| AREA | AGE 10 | 15 | ADULT |
|---|---|---|---|
| A ½ OF HEAD | 5½ | 4½ | 3½ |
| B ½ OF ONE THIGH | 4½ | 4½ | 4½ |
| C ½ OF ONE LEG | 3 | 3½ | 3½ |

% BURN BY AREAS

| | |
|---|---|
| PROBABLE 3RD° BURN | HEAD ... NECK ... BODY ... UP. ARM ... FOREARM ... HANDS ...<br>GENITALS ..... BUTTOCKS ..... THIGHS ..... LEGS ..... FEET ..... |
| TOTAL BURN | HEAD ... NECK ... BODY ... UP. ARM ... FOREARM ... HANDS ...<br>GENITALS ..... BUTTOCKS ..... THIGHS ..... LEGS ..... FEET ..... |

**Figure 3.2** Lund and Browder chart

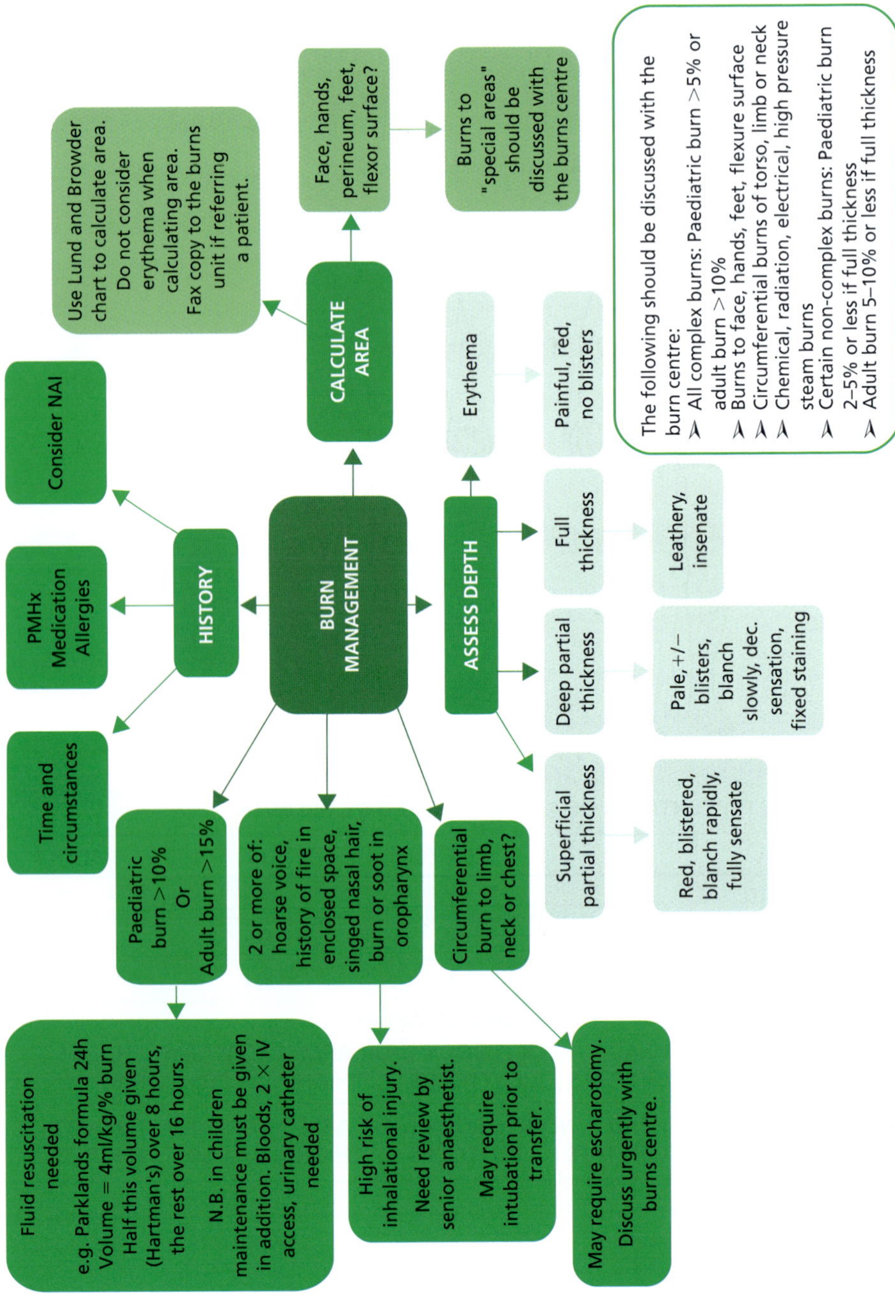


**Figure 3.3** Management of burns

If airway injury is suspected, the patient *must* be reviewed by an anaesthetist before transfer as they may require intubation to secure their airway.

## *Deep circumferential burns*

Deep burns cause skin to lose elasticity. In circumferencial deep burns, the loss of skin elasticity prevents the limb or trunk expanding from the oedema produced by inflamed tissue. Circumferential deep burns in the trunk can lead to reduction in chest wall compliance, which compromises ventilation. Circumferential deep burns of the extremities can compromise circulation of the limb, which can cause tissue ischaemia (Figure 3.4). It therefore may become necessary to release the pressure surgically by making incisions through the burn down to the subcutaneous fat (escharotomies).

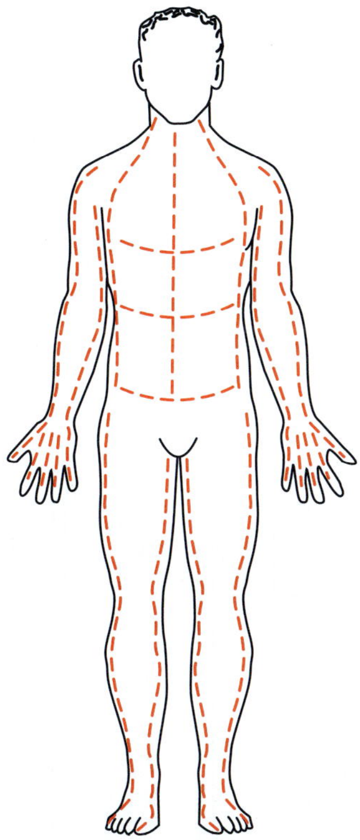

**Figure 3.4** Lines of incision for escharotomies

## *Eyes*

The eyes should always be assessed comprehensively in patients with facial burns to ensure that there is no corneal or globe injury. This often may require a review by an ophthalmologist.

## FLUID RESUSCITATION/PARKLAND FORMULA

Calculate from Time of Burn

**START WITH 0.25mls × % TBSA × weight (kg)**

MLS OF HARTMANNS EACH HOUR (Based on 4mls/Kg/% in 1st 24hrs, with half given in 1st 8 hrs)

**FLUID BALANCE CHART**

Oral fluids are not included in this calculation but should be encouraged

PLEASE COMPLETE THIS CHART WITH ACTUAL VOLUME IN EACH HOUR

N.B. Initial Fluid Treatment should include making up lost time since the burn

| BURN TIME | HOUR 1 | HOUR 2 | HOUR 3 | HOUR 4 |
|---|---|---|---|---|
| Hartmanns (volume) | | | | |
| Other IV Fluids | | | | |
| Oral Fluids | | | | |
| Urine output (mls) | | | | |
| **Analgesia**<br>IV Morphine<br>Other | | | | |

**TRANSFER DETAILS**

Most Senior Doctor to assess patient Grade/Name ____________

Grade of Transferring Person ____________

Time left A&E Department ____________

Mode of Transportation ____________

**OTHER COMMENTS**

____________

## Burns Transfer Information Chart

With thanks to the Burns Unit, The Queen Victoria Hospital NHS Trust, East Grinstead

Name of Hospital ____________ Date/Time arrived A&E ____________

Patients Name ____________ Date of Birth ____________ Weight (kg) ___

**BURN**

Date ____________

Time ____________

Details of First Aid

How accident happened ____________

Other injury (C-Spine?) ____________

Past medical history (Drugs, Allergies, Smoking) ____________

**AIRWAY**

Suspected respiratory injury Yes/No

Soot Yes/No

Singeing Yes/No

Swelling Yes/No

Intubation Grade/Findings

Tube Size ____________ mm

HbCO(%) Time taken

**CIRCULATION**

IV cannula size ____________

Site ____________

**Fluid Resus with Hartmanns (see over)**

Urinary Catheter Yes/No

FBC (Hct) ____________

U&Es ____________

Group and save (send with patient)

Tetanus ____________

**Limb Perfusion** ____________

Escharotomy Performed by ____________

**Full ATLS Secondary Survey**

Performed by ____________

**% Total Body Surface Area Burn (TBSA)**

Be clear and accurate, and do not include erythema (Lund and Browder)

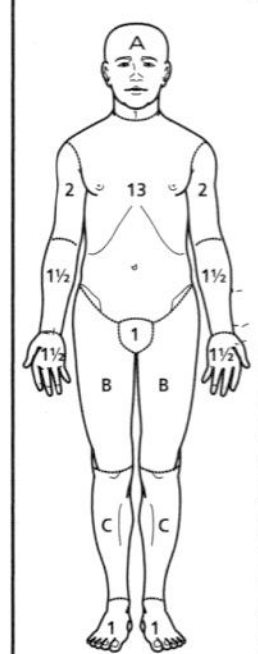


| REGION | % PTL | % FTL |
|---|---|---|
| Head | | |
| Neck | | |
| Ant. Trunk | | |
| Post. Trunk | | |
| Right Arm | | |
| Left Arm | | |
| Buttocks | | |
| Genitalia | | |
| Right Leg | | |
| Left Leg | | |
| Total Burn | | |

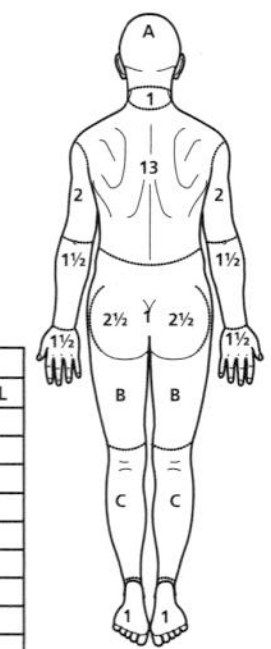


| AREA | Age 0 | 1 | 5 | 10 | 16 | Adult |
|---|---|---|---|---|---|---|
| A = ½ of head | 9.5 | 8.5 | 6.5 | 5.5 | 4.5 | 3.5 |
| B = ½ one thigh | 2.75 | 3.25 | 4 | 4.5 | 4.5 | 4.75 |
| C = ½ one lower leg | 2.5 | 2.5 | 2.75 | 3 | 3.25 | 3.5 |

**Figure 3.5** Transfer form with Lund and Browder chart

## *Fluid resuscitation*

Assessment of burns size is essential for appropriate fluid management. This should be clearly documented on an appropriate Lund and Browder chart (Figure 3.5), taking care to use the appropriate age group for children. Burn size can be best estimated with the charts themselves, 'the rule of nines' or the whole of the patient's palmar surface of the hand as a 1% template.

Fluid resuscitation should be instituted in all patients with a burn size >10% in children and the elderly, or >15% in adults (Figure 3.6).

## *When to admit*

It goes without saying that patients who require ventilatory support or resuscitation fluids require admission, as does any patient with significant facial burns and swelling. Other patients to consider for admission include those with significant hand or genital burns, those who require large dressings, those with infected burns and those who require early surgery.

Any patient who might need to be admitted should be discussed with the on-call consultant burn surgeon. The staff at the burns centre need to be informed of the outcome to ensure effective communication at all levels.

- Use Hartmann's as crystalloid of choice. The formula Maintenance requirements MUST be given AS WELL as Parkland calculations.
- For ease of understanding & clarity, two bags of fluid MUST be used; Hartmann's for fluid resuscitation & Saline for maintenance.
- Described above is only a guide to start therapy. Infusion rate will need to be adjusted according to the response of the patient.
- If urine output not maintained check cannula and catheter. If both OK increase basal fluid rate by 25% OR give bolus of 10ml/kg. If no response repeat. Discuss with senior if still no response. Consider bolus of colloid.
- If urine output is greater than 2 ml/kg/hr re-assess size of burn & weight. If both are accurate then reduce infusion by 25% and re-assess urine output.

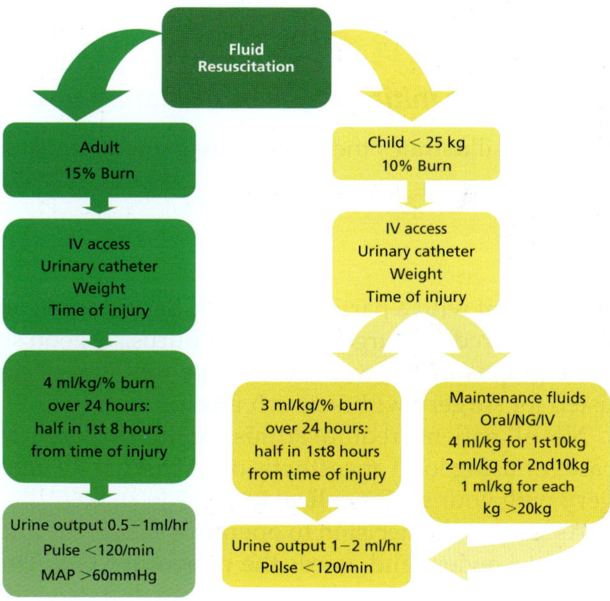


**Figure 3.6** Fluid rescusitation

### *Multidisciplinary support*

Many patients with burn injuries have medical and/or psychiatric problems that require specialist input. Remember that early involvement of physiotherapists, occupational therapists and dieticians in the rehabilitation of patients with burns leads to better outcomes.

## Non-accidental injury

Any inconsistency or change in the history of a child or vulnerable individual with a burn should alert you to the possibility of non-accidental injury. You should also be wary if the history does not seem consistent with the injury sustained. Senior nursing and medical staff need to be made aware of the situation, and the appropriate social services, local paediatricians and physicians and possibly police need to be informed. Accurate documentation, which includes photographs, is essential.

Although you may suspect non-accidental injury, please be aware that the patient must still be treated and those who may be under suspicion of causing the injury may need to be informed of your suspicions. It is essential that all communication is documented, and any action taken needs to be justified. In such a situation, please remember that suspicion does not equal guilt.

Patients with suspected non-accidental injury should not be discharged without the agreement of the relevant paediatricians, social workers, nursing staff and your consultant – even if the burn itself does not need further in-patient treatment.

### *Summary of initial major burn management*

Figure 3.7 illustrates the acute management of major burns.

## Surgery

Any patient with a partial thickness, deep dermal or full thickness burn should be considered for surgery. A senior burns surgeon should review the patient or photographs of the wound to make the final decision. No patient should be listed for surgery without such input.

Not all patients require admission for surgery – some may be treated as day cases or using local anaesthetic only. Discuss the most appropriate time for surgery with your senior colleagues.

As soon as the decision to operate is made, the anaesthetic team must be contacted to review and assess the patient for GA. This often can be done in the dressings clinic before they are admitted. Indeed, if the time between decision and admission is going to be more than a few days, it is important for the

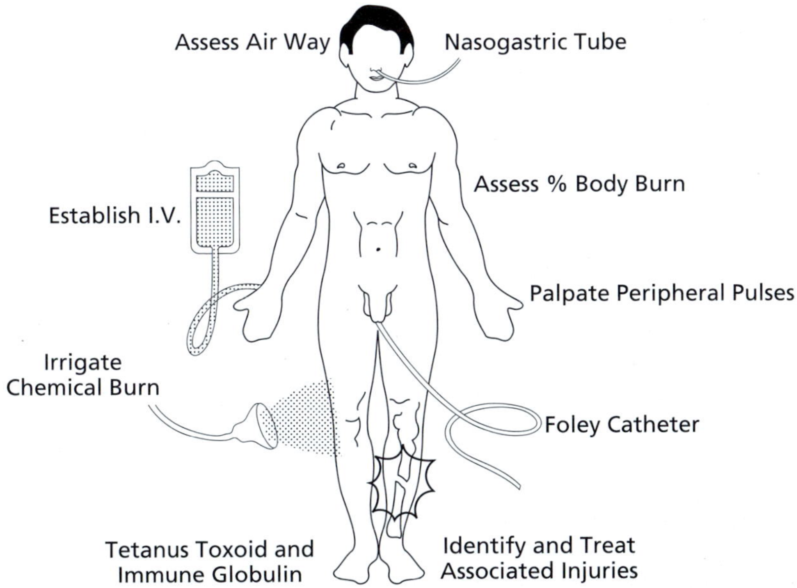


**Figure 3.7** Summary of initial major burns management

anaesthetic team to review the patient *on the day* the decision is made to ensure that the operation is not cancelled on the day.

In general, deeper burns should be treated with surgery as soon as is practical.

## Toxic shock syndrome

Any patient with a burn of any size is at risk of infection of that burn and subsequent sepsis or toxic shock syndrome (TSS). This syndrome is essentially severe septic shock caused by a bacterial endotoxin, most commonly produced by *Staphylococcus aureus*.

Toxic shock syndrome is diagnosed on the basis of a high index of clinical suspicion, as no laboratory test is available to confirm the diagnosis. A significant increase in the level of antibody against toxic shock syndrome toxin (TSST)-1 in serum in association with clinical manifestation is strong retrospective support for the diagnosis.

**Criteria for diagnosis of toxic shock syndrome**

- Temperature >38.9°C
- Erythematous rash
- Hypotension and poor peripheral perfusion

Children are at particular risk of TSS. If you are called to see a patient with a burn who is feverish and unwell, your first consideration should be sepsis or TSS. Take a full history and examine the patient to determine the source of sepsis. A full set of blood tests is required, including blood cultures. Take this condition very seriously, as affected patients can deteriorate very quickly. Establish wide-calibre intravenous access. Start fluid resuscitation, discuss with the microbiology department and involve your senior colleagues (registrar, anaesthetist, microbiologist) immediately.

## Pharmacy guidelines for burns

Table 3.2 summarizes the pharmacy guidelines for burns.

**Table 3.2** Pharmacy guidelines for burns.

| Treatment | Directions |
|---|---|
| Fluid resuscitation (Parkland's formula) (if burn >15% body surface area in adults) | • 4 ml of Hartmann's solution per kg per percentage body surface area of burn in first 24 hours; half of this volume to be given in first eight hours<br>• Aim for urine output > 0.5 ml/kg/hour, heart rate <120 per minute and calm, lucid patient<br>• Dose for fluid resuscitation in children: 3 mg per kg per percentrage burn, but maintenance fluid also should be given |
| Inhalation injury | • Hourly nebules as below<br>• Use preprinted sheets<br>• Nebulized salbutamol 2.5–5 mg every four hours<br>• Nebulized acetylcysteine 20% 3 ml every four hours<br>• Nebulized sodium bicarbonate 2.1% 2.5–5 ml every two hours<br>• Salbutamol must be given before first acetylcysteine nebule<br>• Anaesthetist must be involved |
| Stress ulcer prophylaxis | • Ranitidine 50 mg intravenously every eight hours until tolerating enteral feed |
| Prokinetics | • First-line metoclopramide: 10–20 mg four times daily intravenously, orally or by nasogastric tube<br>• Second-line erythromycin: 250 mg every 6–8 hours orally, by nasogastric tube or intravenously |
| Itching | • Antihistamines: chlorpheniramine 4 mg every 4–6 hours or hydroxyzine 25 mg at night, increasing to four times daily*<br>• 0.5% menthol in aqueous cream also can be applied |
| Flammercerium (silver sulfadiazine and cerium nitrate cream) | • Used on partial thickness, deep dermal and full thickness burns (unlicensed product)<br>• Decreases bacterial growth |
| Heparin prophylaxis for deep vein thrombosis | • Tinzaparin, as per local guidelines |
| Heparin treatment for pulmonary embolism or deep vein thrombosis | • Unfractionated heparin, as per local guidelines |

*Can cause sedation.

# Facial trauma

Facial trauma comes under the remit of plastic surgeons, ear, nose and throat surgeons, ophthalmic surgeons and oral and maxillofacial surgeons. The way in which facial trauma cases are divided between these surgeons depends on each specialty's availability and local expertise, which will vary from hospital to hospital. Units with craniofacial or head and neck interests will tend to take a greater breadth of facial trauma cases than others. In contrast, if your hospital has maxillofacial surgeons, you may find they take all facial traumas – even lip lacerations. Find out your unit's exact policy from your colleagues. Generally, however, nasal fractures, septal haematomas and sometimes pinna haematomas go to ear, nose and throat surgeons, whereas facial and mandibular fractures and oral trauma go to maxillofacial surgeons.

It is important to perform a thorough examination in cases of facial trauma so that important diagnoses are not missed.

**Diagnoses/signs that can be overlooked in patients with facial trauma**

- Airway compromise
- Serious head and neck injuries
- Visual impairment
- Diplopia
- Blow-out fractures
- Ocular foreign bodies
- Septal haematomas
- Parotid duct lacerations
- Facial nerve palsies
- Malocclusion
- Facial and mandibular fractures
- Fractures of the skull base
- Deafness

Before accepting a referral for a facially injured patient from the emergency department, make sure that facial trauma is their only problem and that they do not have other injuries that would not be appropriate for a plastic surgeon to manage. You should therefore make sure that serious head injury has been excluded and confirm that the cervical spine is clear through appropriate radiology. If the patient does have other injuries, insist that the referring doctor makes successful referrals to other specialties. The principle is to avoid having a patient with a simple facial laceration who then turns out to have a serious head injury, a compromised airway and an open tibia fracture admitted solely under your care. Discuss such cases early with the other relevant specialties, make sure the patient goes to the appropriate ward and coordinate surgery so that the facial trauma can be addressed at the same time as other procedures.

Most facial trauma is minor and can wait until the next day for surgery. Some cases, however, may need urgent surgery and should be discussed with your registrar straight away; this includes patients with airway involvement, Le Fort facial fractures, uncontrolled bleeding, reduced visual acuity, gross wound contamination, penetrating neck wounds and polytrauma. Septal and pinna haematomas need urgent incision and drainage to prevent necrosis of the underlying cartilage.

## History

The purpose of taking the patient's history is to elucidate the nature of the injury and therefore the likelihood of head injury, foreign bodies, nerve/ducts damage and contamination and the need for facial views. Make a note of the patient's age, sex and occupation and gauge their attitude to cosmesis. For example, you may be able to stitch up a large facial laceration on an elderly male labourer in the emergency department, but a much smaller laceration in a 25-year-old female model may be more appropriate for your registrar.

## Examination

Initially, you should follow the principles of advanced trauma life support (ATLS) because of the association with polytrauma. Table 3.3 shows a suggested scheme for a full facial examination (see also Figure 3.8).

## Lip lacerations

You can repair uncontaminated and straightforward lip lacerations yourself in the emergency department. Use local infiltration with LA and adrenaline or infraorbital nerve blocks for upper lip lacerations. Mark the vermillion border carefully before injecting anaesthetic, as the swelling may distort the anatomy and lead to incorrect alignment. Closure is in three layers – mucosa, muscle and skin (although muscle and mucosa can be sutured as one layer if difficult). For the skin, use 5/0 or 6/0 nylon and place the first two stitches above and below the vermillion border. Discharge the patient with oral antibiotics and ask them to return in five days so that the sutures can be removed and the wound checked.

**Table 3.3** Suggested scheme for a full facial examination.

| Examination | Points of note |
|---|---|
| Airway | |
| Cervical spine | |
| Glasgow coma scale (GCS) | Eyes – 4, Verbal – 5, Motor – 6 |
| General facial appearance | • Asymmetry (swelling, fractures)<br>• Depressions (maxilla, Le Fort fractures)<br>• Zygoma fractures |
| Eyes | • Shape of pupils<br>• Globe rupture<br>• Subconjunctival haemorrhage (skull fractures)<br>• Enopthalmos (sunken eye)<br>• Hypoglobus (globe lower than normal side)<br>• Problems on ophthalmoscopy (foreign bodies, retinal detachment)<br>• Pupils equal, round, reactive to light and accommodation (PERRLA)<br>• Decreased visual acuity<br>• Diplopia<br>• Damage to lacrimal gland or duct (reduced tears)<br>• Pain suggests corneal injury |
| Nose | • Deviation<br>• Obstructed breathing<br>• Fractures<br>• Septal haematoma (red swelling filling whole of one or both nostrils) |
| Mouth | • Lip lacerations<br>• Teeth malocclusion<br>• Airway compromise<br>• Bleeding |
| Facial sensation | • Decreased sensation over maxilla implies damage to infraorbital nerve from fracture of maxilla<br>• Numbness of lower lip implies damage to inferior alveolar nerve suggesting mandibular fracture |
| Facial nerve | • Any degree of facial palsy mandates exploration |
| Palpation | • Bony tenderness or steps |
| Facial laceration | • Note position:<br>  ○ Does it cross nerve/duct territories – i.e. will it need proper exploration in theatre?<br>  ○ Does it cross important aesthetic structures – vermillion border, eyebrows, nasolabial fold?<br>  ○ How deep is it? |

## Facial lacerations

You will be called to see many facial lacerations, most of which are minor. Clean superficial wounds with edges that are not jagged and are not associated with nerve or duct injury need minimal debridement and can be sutured, fixed

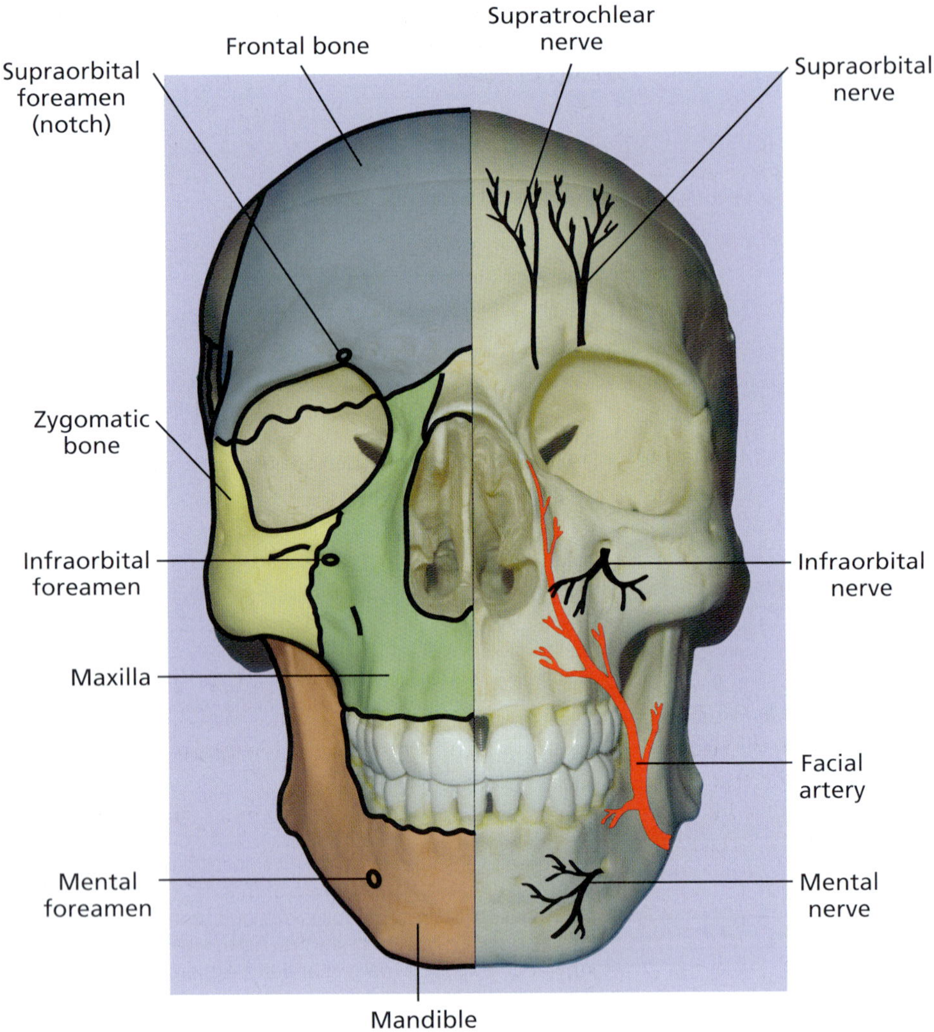


**Figure 3.8** Facial bones and important structures in the face

with sterile strips or glued in the emergency department. Use local infiltration with adrenaline. Use interrupted nylon for the skin. Close the muscle separately. Sutures must be removed five days after they are applied or they will leave marks. Give the patient oral antibiotics if necessary. The wound can be checked in the dressing clinic when the sutures are removed, unless it is particularly complicated or disfiguring, in which case formal outpatient assessment is warranted.

## Facial fractures

Obtain facial radiographs if you suspect foreign bodies (especially in relation to the globe), if there is a history of blunt trauma or if you find bony tenderness or swelling on examination. Ask for a postero-anterior view and a Caldwell view (postero-anterior view with head extended 23°) and an orthopantogram (OPG) to demonstrate mandibular fractures. Facial views are difficult to interpret, so ask a registrar to go through a system with you. Essentially, however, you should trace the superior and inferior margins of the maxilla from one side to the other looking for steps or breaks in continuity and then repeat for the orbital margins. Examine all the sinuses for fluid levels. Look carefully at the condyles for mandibular fractures.

Common fractures are of the mandible, zygoma, orbit, maxilla, nasal and frontal sinus. Maxilla fractures are graded into Le Fort 1, 2 and 3 and demonstrate increasing craniofacial dysjunction. These are high-energy injuries. Often more than one fracture is present.

If you find a facial fracture, always make sure the airway is not compromised. If it is, you must act immediately: sit the patient up, give them high-flow oxygen and fast bleep the anaesthetist and your registrar. The patient will need a definitive airway (orotracheal intubation or surgical airway), so proceed as per the ATLS protocol. Remember that nasotracheal intubation is contraindicated in facial fractures because of the risk of the tube passing down a false passage.

Most facial fractures need operative intervention because of the deformity and functional impairment they cause. Orbital fractures will need to be imaged with computed tomography (CT). The registrar should see the patient and will want to see all the radiographs and subsequent computed tomograms. All but the most minor fractures will warrant admission of the affected patient. At night, it would be best to admit the patient and prepare for surgery the next day. If there is any airway, optical or neurological compromise, the patient has an associated head injury, the patient has multiple injuries or the patient will be going to theatre with other specialties that night, inform the registrar on admission.

**Key management points**

- Admit all but simple facial lacerations
- Consider airway and other injuries
- Look for ocular and nerve injuries and facial fractures
- Check for dental occlusion
- Consider computed tomography and early senior review if fracture present

# Lower limb trauma

You will be referred cases of lower limb trauma by the emergency department and orthopaedic team. The bulk of this work will entail pretibial lacerations and open fractures, mainly of the tibia. Clarify with your registrar whether or not your unit accepts lower limb trauma referrals, as some units do not.

The role of plastic surgeons in lower limb trauma is to restore soft tissue cover. In the case of pretibial lacerations, this may mean split-skin grafting. In the case of open pretibial fractures, it will mean anything from direct closure to split-skin grafts, local flaps, perforator flaps and free flaps.

## Pretibial lacerations

Patients with pretibial lacerations that need plastic surgical input tend to be elderly and female. This is because even quite minor trauma can lead to large wounds in the oedematous leg with fragile skin. The poor quality of skin in this

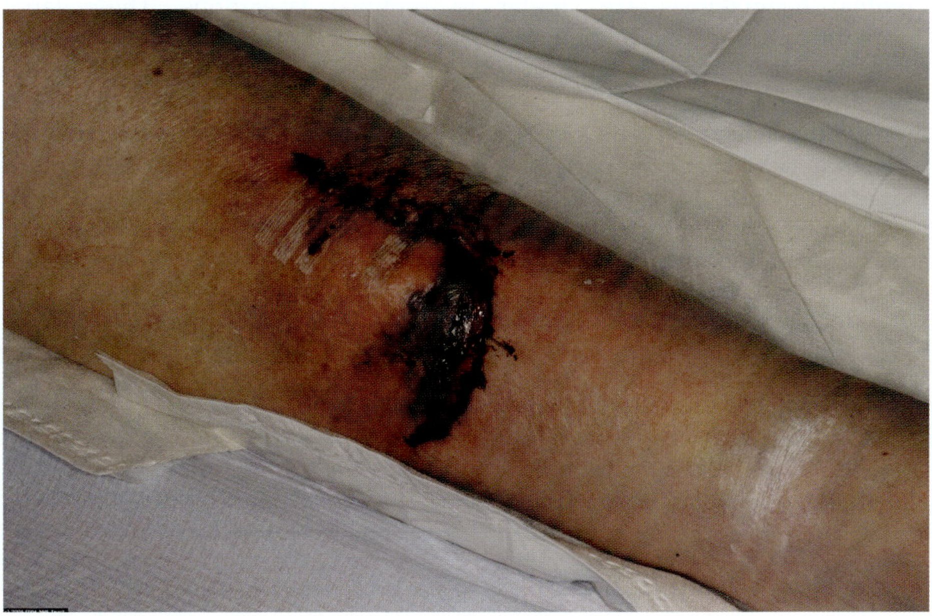

**Figure 3.9** Pretibial laceration

area means that these wounds cannot be simply sutured closed in the emergency department, because the stitches will tend to pull through and the skin flaps die, especially those with a narrow base. In the case of small pretibial lacerations, simple debridement and regular dressing changes in the dressing clinic may suffice, with the proviso that these wounds can take weeks to heal. For larger wounds, debridement and split-skin grafting is the preferred option, as skin cover is achieved much sooner, which reduces the risks of infection and delayed mobilization.

When taking a referral for a patient with a pretibial laceration, question closely about the cause. The injury may have been sustained as a result of an acute medical problem that needs more urgent attention. In such cases, the wound can be treated as and when the medical condition has been addressed. As long as these wounds are clean, operations can safely be delayed for a few days.

Patients with pretibial lacerations may need to be admitted; if they are referred at night, this can be safely done the next morning. They will need full blood count and group and screen and other investigations depending on their medical status. They should be booked for a GA, although they may require spinal anaesthesia if medically unfit. If you suspect this to be the case, involve your anaesthetic colleagues early.

## Pretibial haematomas

Pretibial haematomas are similar to pretibial lacerations. These large haematomas are caused by blunt and often minor trauma and, again, usually occur in elderly women who are taking warfarin. The toxic effects of the haematoma breaking down causes the skin overlying the haematoma to die, so these wounds need the same debridement and cover as pretibial lacerations. It is mandatory to check the patient's international normalized ratio (INR), stop the warfarin and add heparin prophylaxis. If the patient is receiving warfarin for anything other than atrial fibrillation, you are advised to confirm the correct anticoagulant regimen with a haematologist or cardiologist, as appropriate.

**Key management points**

- Clean and dress in the emergency department
- Address underlying cause
- Admit for wound debridement and split skin grafting under GA
- Full blood count and group and save (with or without INR)

## Open tibial fractures

In patients with open tibial fractures, obtain a full history because these injuries are often associated with high-energy impact and polytrauma.

You should find out the following:

- Age
- Mechanism of injury
- Time since injury
- Time since last food/drink
- Presence of other injuries
- Current resuscitation status
- Details of fracture
- Status of limb – vascular and neurological; presence of compartment syndrome
- Previous medical history
- Premorbid mobility
- Orthopaedic team's plan.

The ideal way for these injuries to be managed is through joint care by orthopaedic and plastic surgeons, with consultant involvement from presentation. If you are referred a patient with an open tibial fracture, therefore, you must discuss them with your registrar before any transfer.

Usually, however, transfer and sometimes referral of these patients occurs after the orthopaedic surgeons have undertaken (usually external) fixation of the fracture. Collect the same information before transfer and again discuss the case with your registrar. In this scenario, your senior colleagues may request certain investigations, such as arteriograms, before transfer.

On admission, obtain a full and detailed history from the patient and notes, paying particular attention to the mechanism of injury, and what investigations and procedures have occurred since the injury. Collect the investigations together, especially the radiographs, arteriograms and any other imaging of the limb. Examine the patient carefully for other injuries according to the principles of ATLS. Examine the limb for:

- colour
- capillary refill
- compartment syndrome (pain not in keeping with the injury, pain on passive movement)
- sensation
- movement
- all pulses
- temperature.

If there is any suspicion of ischaemia or compartment syndrome, notify your registrar immediately.

Do not simply book the patient for theatre as normal, as your consultant will want to see the patient first in order to decide on the correct procedure. Furthermore, the procedure may be performed on an elective list rather than a trauma list.

You should work the patient up as if they were going to a have a free flap operation, which may be the case. You should arrange for a full blood count, urea and electrolytes, group and screen (including arranging four units of whole blood if the patient is undergoing a free-flap operation), relevant imaging and any other investigations dictated by the patient's medical status.

Joint plastics and orthopaedics guidelines suggest that wounds ideally should be closed within five days.

**Key management points**

- Admit for GA after discussion with senior colleagues
- Examine the patient for other injuries and the limb for ischaemia and compartment syndrome
- Full blood count, urea and electrolytes and group and save (with or without blood cross-match)

# 4

# Miscellaneous

The chapters in this section are a guide to the other problems you will encounter when on call for plastic surgery. This section also includes information on performing minor operations, as you may be expected to perform these lists alone.

# Ward problems

## Free flaps

A thorough handover at the start of a shift is important. Ideally you need to see a free flap early, so you can assess any change if you are called to review. Assessment of free flaps while on-call is very common, so it is important to have a system that works for you. Always inform your senior colleagues early if you are concerned about compromise of free flaps. Although the first 48 hours after the operation are the critical time for a free flap to survive, remember that a free flap can become compromised during the procedure and until five days or more postoperatively.

Assessment involves finding out about the type of free flap and reading the operative notes to see if there were any problems in theatre or if there are any special postoperative instructions. When seeing a patient with a free flap, check the flap and the patient (Table 4.1). Examination of the patient and the flap begins with monitoring vital signs and assessing trends since surgery. Always consider intrinsic and extrinsic factors that can influence flap survival. The flap may be compromised if the patient is hypotensive, hypovolaemic, hypoxic or otherwise unwell. The flap itself may be compromised

**Table 4.1** Checking a patient with a free flap.

| Patient | Flap |
|---|---|
| • Is the patient well?<br>• Heart rate and blood pressure<br>• Colour<br>• Respiratory rate<br>• Oxygen saturations<br>• Urine output (must be at least 1 ml/kg)<br>• Fluid input and output<br>• Receiving anticoagulants or intravenous dextrans<br>• Postoperative haemoglobin/haematocrit | • Flap chart<br>  ○ Change in colour<br>  ○ Pale – arterial problem<br>  ○ Blue – venous problem<br>  ○ Fixed purple staining – necrosis<br>• Capillary refill – should be two seconds, reduced if poor perfusion, brisk if venous congestion<br>• Temperature – body temperature is normal, cold if compromised<br>• Is this a global change or regional/zonal change?* |

*A global change may be amenable to improving a patient's general health and perfusion, whereas a zonal change implies problems with anastamosis that may require a visit to theatre.

because of arterial or venous components as well as a haematoma. Free flaps are often pale in the hours after surgery, but they should be warm, soft and have a normal capillary refill. They should bleed bright red oxygenated blood when pierced with a needle. A white flap with loss of any of the former characteristics indicates acute arterial compromise. A blue, swollen flap with a brisk capillary refill that oozes dark blood when pierced with a needle indicates venous congestion. In both of these situations, you should call the registrar to see the patient *immediately* as the flap will die unless promptly salvaged in the operating theatre. Keep the patient nil by mouth and prepare them for an emergency return to theatre.

**Key management points**

- Read operative notes
- Check observation charts
  - Pulse
  - Blood pressure
  - Urine output
  - Temperature
- Examine patient
- Examine flap:
  - Colour (zonal/global, pale/dark blue)
  - Temperature
  - Capillary refill time
  - Doppler if vessel area marked perioperatively

Figure 4.1 illustrates a venous congested free flap. Figure 4.2 illustrates arterial insufficiency and zonal necrosis. Figure 4.3 illustrates reversible zonal compromise; unlike in Figure 4.2, the arterial insufficiency has been detected early and therefore can be reversed to salvage the flap.

Fixed staining due to necrosis is usually partial and at the edge of the flap most distal to the pedicle. The timing of this fixed staining is crucial. If it appears acutely it indicates flap ischaemia. If it appears gradually over days, and the attending team will usually be aware of it, so it does not need immediate action. If the flap is compromised, however, inform your senior colleague, because the flap will need to be salvaged through surgery as soon as possible. You should prepare the patient for theatre by arranging blood tests, 4–6 crossmatched units of blood, consent and marking and by informing the anaesthetist and theatre staff.

Always inform a senior if you are unsure. They will not be upset with an unnecessary call, but they will be upset if they are not informed of a compromised flap that could have been saved by early treatment.

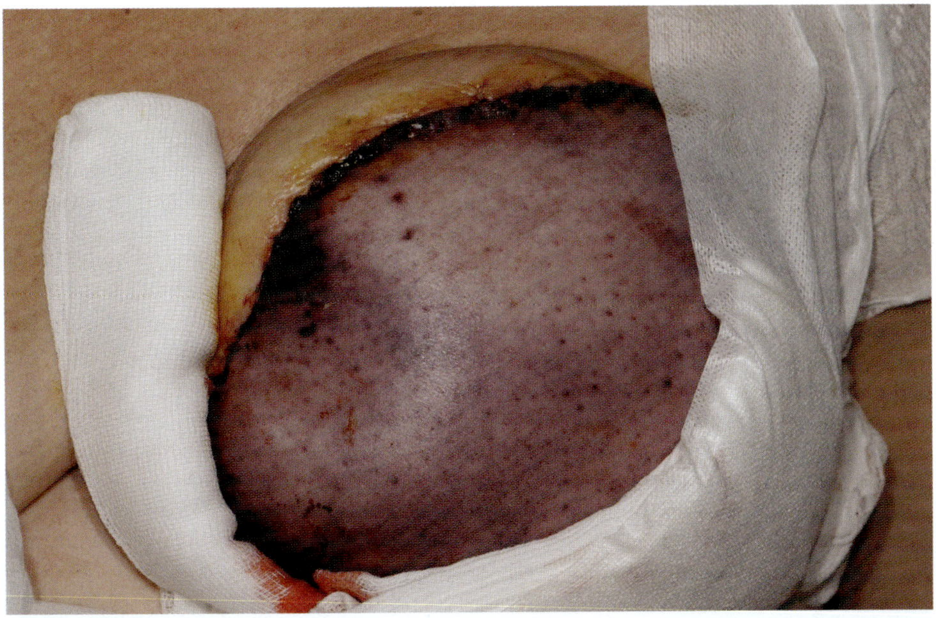

**Figure 4.1** Globally congested free flap

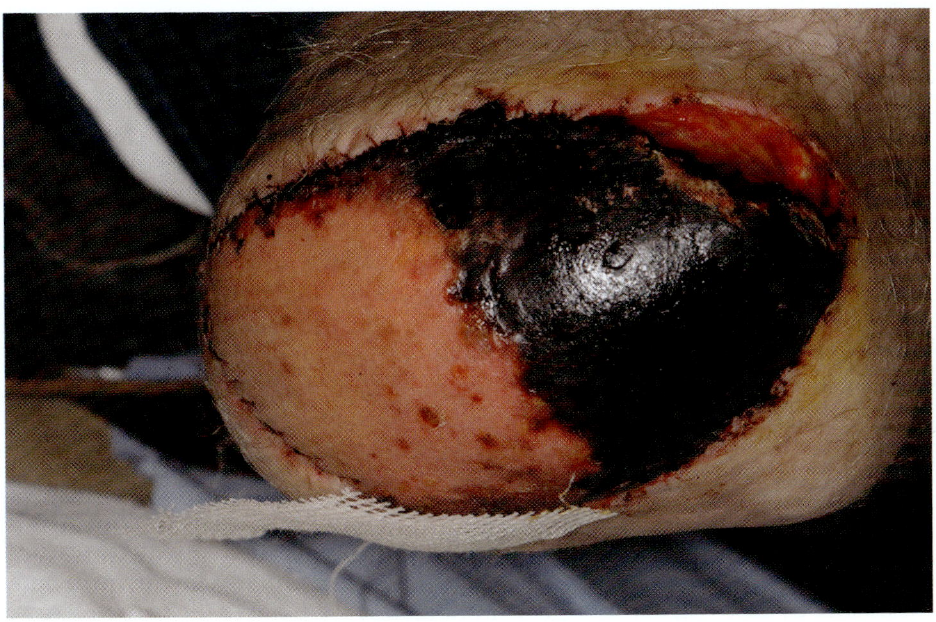

**Figure 4.2** Irreversible zonal necrosis of free flap

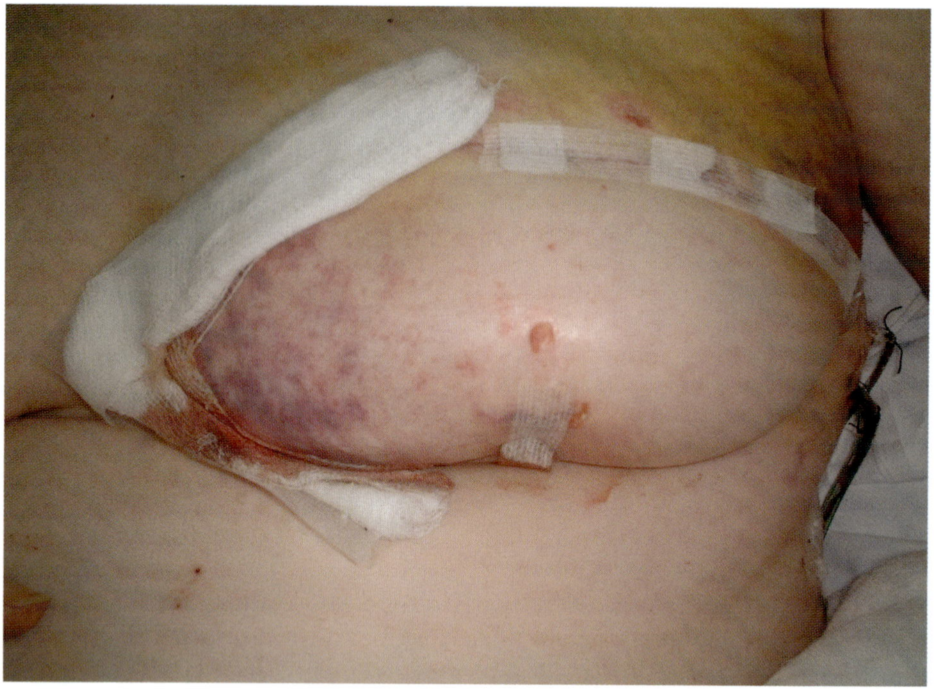

**Figure 4.2** Reversible zonal compromise

## Compartment syndrome

Compartment syndrome is a surgical emergency that needs immediate surgical intervention. It is defined as a rise in pressure in a fascia/bone-enclosed compartment, which is sufficient to impair perfusion. In plastic surgery, this mainly refers to muscle compartments. It is most frequent in patients with trauma of the hand, forearm or lower limb, especially when the patient has fractures or crush injuries. Nevertheless, compartment syndrome also can occur after elective surgery and can be caused by casts that are too tight (see below).

The clinical features of compartment syndrome are unexpectedly severe pain not relieved by normal analgesia, numbness (first dorsal webspace numbness is characteristic of lower limb anterior compartment syndrome), pain on passive extension of the muscle compartment in question, reduced capillary refill and absent pulses (end stage).

If you have the slightest suspicion of compartment syndrome, ask your registrar to see the patient immediately – you will never be criticized for misdiagnosing compartment syndrome, but you will be hung, drawn and quartered if you miss it. Alert the registrar, anaesthetist and theatre, and prepare the patient for theatre as they will need surgery immediately – whatever the time of day or night.

Some units use compartment pressure monitoring, but if the index of suspicion is high, time should not be wasted before decompression.

**Consent for treatment of compartment syndrome**

- Infection, haematoma, GA
- Two wounds the length of the forearm or leg or several incisions on the hand
- Immediate or delayed split-skin grafting of these wounds or delayed direct closure

**Key management points**

Look for:

- pain out of synch with the nature of injury
- pain on passive movement

## Painful casts

Postoperatively, painful casts are a common problem on the ward. If you are called to see a patient with a painful cast, check what operation they have had and when – this will tell you the implication of taking off the cast, and will confirm whether or not the surgeon has given special instructions such as 'Do not take off the cast without calling me'! Assess how much pain the patient is in and what analgesia they have had. Answer the following questions: Does the patient have more than the expected postoperative pain? Is the limb elevated? Does the cast feel too tight? Does the patient have numbness of the digits? If it is possible to flex and extend the digits passively without compromising the surgery, do so and note whether or not it is painful.

If the patient has more than the expected pain and it is not responding to analgesia or you suspect compartment syndrome, carefully remove the cast with the plaster saw in such a way that it can be reassembled in the same position when wrapped in a bandage. If the pain is eased by removal of the cast, it was probably too tight. Put the cast back on, but not as tightly, with a bandage. Elevate the limb and arrange for a new, looser cast. If the pain is not relieved, remove the dressings to check for a haematoma. If a haematoma is present, alert the registrar and arrange for evacuation of the haematoma.

If the patient has compartment syndrome, they will have a tense, tender hand or forearm, pain on passive movement of the digits, numbness and, if prolonged, reduced capillary refill and pulses. This is a major emergency (see page 118).

**Key management points**

- Check operative notes
- Check analgesia
- Assess tightness of cast
- Assess swelling of the limb
- Look for haematoma or signs of compartment syndrome
- Elevate limb, arrange suitable analgesia and release cast if necessary to relieve tightness
- Review

## Haematomas

A postoperative haematoma, which is recognized as a tense, dark, painful swelling, as a rule needs to be drained urgently, so do call your registrar at any time. Urgent surgery is needed not only to stop the bleeding but also to prevent damage to surrounding tissues or flaps caused by the pressure. For example, a haematoma will compromise a free flap, the pedicle to the nipple in a breast reduction or the median nerve in carpal tunnel decompression, and the breakdown products will necrotize any overlying skin or graft. Removal of one or two sutures to express a small old haematoma a few days down the line may be acceptable; however, the patient needs to go back to theatre in the case of an acute postoperative haematoma. Arrange a group and save, and crossmatch for patients with a free flap.

**Consent for evacuation of haematoma**

- Infection, further haematoma, scars, GA
- Loss of free flap, loss of nipple (bilateral breast reduction)

**Key management points**

- Check operative notes
- Check observations
- Examine patient for tense swelling or tenderness
- Review analgesia
- Importantly, do not forget that patients may lose a significant amount of blood

# Dressings clinic

You will hear the question, 'What dressing do you want on that?', time and time again. Knowledge of the correct type of dressing is important – not only during your time in the plastics department but throughout your medical career. You will be asked to review wounds, and prescription of the correct type of dressing can make a great deal of difference to healing time. Table 4.2 lists commonly used dressings, ointments and creams and describes their action on wounds. Many of these dressings are interchangeable and different units and consultants have their own preferences – due to experience, cost issues or local guidelines – so find out what your unit uses. To start with, do not make unilateral decisions, especially when dressing acute wounds such as burns. Always consult with your registrar or consultant and take the advice of the nurse in charge of the unit – they have been dressing wounds for years!

**Guidelines when called to the dressing clinic to look at a wound**

- Wound infection – will require oral/intravenous antibiotics and possibly surgical debridement
- Wound dehiscence – if small, may be treated conservatively to heal by secondary intention; if significant, may require closure
- Stitch abscess – sutures need to be removed in dressing clinic, which may require local anaesthesia; may also need a course of antibiotics
- Seroma – if small, can be managed conservatively; if significant, will need drainage with needle and syringe (caution with flaps, be aware of anastamoses)
- Haematoma – will need evacuation unless small
- Graft failure – look for underlying cause; when treated, reassess for regrafting or other means of cover

If in doubt always consult your senior colleagues.

**Table 4.2** Properties of different dressings, ointments and creams.

| Dressing | Properties |
|---|---|
| Mepitel | • Non-adhesive dressing<br>• Used for up to a week<br>• Expensive |
| Jelonet | • Non-adhesive dressing<br>• Used for 24 hours<br>• Relatively cheap |
| Duoderm | • Hydrocolloid<br>• Absorbs water and forms a gel<br>• Used for non-oozing wounds |
| Telfa | • Non-adhesive dressing<br>• Cheap |
| Vacutex | • Has capillary refill action<br>• Promotes granulation<br>• Good for sloughly necrotic tissue<br>• Sometimes placed on top of Jelonet/Mepitel to prevent adhesion to wounds |
| Intrasite | • Hydrogel<br>• Moistens and softens wounds |
| Calcium gluconate | • Used in burns with hydrofluoric acid (an emergency*) |
| Bactroban (mupirocin 2%) | • Antimicrobial, especially covering Gram-positive organisms, including methicillin-resistant *Staphylococcus aureus*!<br>• Used in erythamatous burns but needs changing every 24 hours |
| Metrotop | • Contains metronidazole<br>• Used when anaerobic infections suspected – for example, in patients with diabetes<br>• Also moistens wounds |
| Betadine | • Antiseptic<br>• Tendency to dry up wounds and stick, so if you are applying a betadine-soaked gauze, use Mepitel or Jelonet underneath to prevent the gauze sticking to the wound |
| Unguentum M | • Moisturizer<br>• Very good for wounds that are dry and itchy! |
| Furacine | • 0.2% nitrofurazone (yellow)<br>• Used in partial thickness burns with Mepitel or Jelonet<br>• Anti-Gram-positive properties<br>• Tendency to dry up wounds |
| Flamazine (1% silver sulfadiazine) | • Anti-Gram-negative properties, especially *Pseudomonas,* and is relatively broad spectrum<br>• Covers infections with staphylococci<br>• Moistens wounds<br>• Lifts up scabs and scars<br>• Helps separation between eschars and wounds<br>• Can cause transient decrease in white cell count<br>• Usually changed on a daily basis but can be left up to 48 hours |
| Hydrocortisone/Terracortil | • Used for overgranulation (silver nitrate sticks also can be used) |

*Even a 1–2% burn with hydrofluoric acid can cause life-threatening hypocalcaemia.

# Minor operations

You almost certainly will have your own minor operations list. Such lists are mainly for the excision biopsies of basal cell carcinomas, squamous cell carcinomas, suspected melanomas and treatment of epidermal cysts, seborrhoeic keratoses and recalcitrant solar keratoses.

Tumorous lesions should be excised with the full thickness of skin plus a layer of subcutaneous fat, which, in areas of thin skin such as the face, will mean excision to the depth of the superficial fascia. You therefore must be aware of superficial nerves – for example, the temporal branch of the facial nerve. If a lesion is in the area of a nerve (which is particularly likely for lesions on the face), preoperatively examine and document sensation and movements. Warn the patient that it may be necessary to sacrifice the nerve. If you do encounter a nerve, try and preserve it. If the tumour and its margins cannot be removed without sacrificing the nerve, it is acceptable to do so unless the lesion is benign.

Before surgery, look in the notes for any instructions about excision margins and whether or not you should close the wound directly with a local flap or full thickness skin graft. Do not use local flaps unnecessarily after excising potential tumours because a flap may complicate re-excision if excision is incomplete.

Prepare the patient as you would in theatre. Draw and measure the excision margins. Locally infiltrate with local anaesthetic and adrenaline except in the vicinity of the digits, penis and nipples (structures with end arteries), although this is now a contentious area.

After closure, dress the wound with sterile strips and an absorbent adhesive dressing. Tell the patient to expect some bleeding. Give patients with ulcerated lesions a course of oral antibiotics as they are particularly prone to wound infections.

The literature on excision margins is complex and the consultant will usually indicate required margins, but Table 4.3 provides a guide. Table 4.4 shows suggested sutures and follow-up.

**Table 4.3** Suggested excision margins

| Lesion | Suggested excision margin |
|---|---|
| Suspected melanoma | 2 mm |
| Basal cell carcinoma | 3 mm |
| Squamous cell carcinoma | 4 mm |

**Table 4.4** Sutures and follow-up.

| Body site | Dermal suture | Superfical suture | Removal of sutures |
|---|---|---|---|
| Face | 6/0 single filament absorbable e.g. Monocryl | 6/0 non-absorbable single filament e.g. nylon | 5 days |
| Back | 3/0 single filament absorbable | 4/0–5/0 non-absorbable or subcuticular absorbable | 2 weeks |
| Limbs and torso | 4/0 single filament absorbable | 5/0 non-absorbable or subcuticular absorbable | 2 weeks |
| Hands | – | 5/0 non-absorbable | 2 weeks |

# Index

page numbers in bold refer to tables